Practice and Research in Social Work

Although postmodernist theories have been thoroughly analysed in sociology and to some extent, in social policy, by addressing current debates in social work *Practice and Research in Social Work* is the first book to appraise key issues in the contested fields of postmodernism and feminism.

With contributors from the UK, Australia, South Africa and Canada, the chapters cover issues such as:

- postmodernity and postmodern feminism
- disability
- a postmodern perspective on professional ethics
- deconstructing and reconstructing professional expertise
- researching mothers' violence
- profeminist men's narratives
- representations of families.

Practice and Research in Social Work will be essential reading for students of social work and social policy.

Barbara Fawcett and **Brid Featherstone** are Senior Lecturers in Social Work at the University of Bradford; **Jan Fook** is Foundation Professor of Social Work at Deakin University, Geelong, Australia; **Amy Rossiter** is Senior Lecturer at Atkinson College, University of York, Ontario, Canada.

Practice and Research in Social Work

Postmodern feminist perspectives

Edited by Barbara Fawcett, Brid Featherstone, Jan Fook and Amy Rossiter

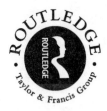

London and New York

First published 2000
by Routledge
11 New Fetter Lane, London EC4P 4EE

Simultaneously published in the USA and Canada
by Routledge
29 West 35th Street, New York, NY 10001

Routledge is an imprint of the Taylor & Francis Group

Typeset in Garamond by Taylor & Francis Books Ltd
Printed and bound in Great Britain by MPG Books Ltd, Bodmin

British Library Cataloguing in Publication Data
A catalogue record for this book is available from the British Library

Library of Congress Cataloging in Publication Data
Practice and research in social work: postmodern feminist perspectives
Edited by Barbara Fawcett et *al*. Includes bibliographical
references and index. 1. Social service. 2. Social service – Research.
3. Postmodernism – Social aspects. 4. Feminist theory. 5. Feminism.
I. Fawcett, Barbara.
HV41.P65 2000   99–31189
362.3'2–dc21   CIP

ISBN 0–415–19511–X (hbk)
ISBN 0–415–19512–8 (pbk)

Contents

Contributors

Vivienne Bozalek is a lecturer at the University of the Western Cape, an historically black institution which has had progressive policies for the past decade. She teaches in the Social Work Department and Gender Studies Unit. Her research interests are in research methodology, and women and social policy.

Barbara Fawcett is Senior Lecturer in Social Work at the University of Bradford. She has published widely in the areas of feminism, postmodernism and social work and is currently carrying out research into feminism postmodernism and disability.

Brid Featherstone is Senior Lecturer in Social Work at the University of Bradford. She has published in the areas of gender relations and violence, and feminist theory generally. She is co-editor with B. Fawcett, J. Hearn and C. Toft of *Violence and Gender Relations* (Sage, 1996) and with W. Hollway of *Mothering and Ambivalence* (Routledge, 1997).

Jan Fook has taught in social work and welfare courses around Australia for the last fifteen years. She is currently Professor of Social Work at Deakin University, Geelong, Australia. Most of her published research work is on social work practice, and she has published on radical and feminist social work, rural social work, and social work expertise. She is the author of *Radical Casework; A Theory of Practice* (Allen and Unwin, 1993) which is used widely in Australia and Canada, and also in the UK, New Zealand and Asia. She is also the editor of *The Reflective Researcher: Social Workers' Theories of Practice Research* (Allen and Unwin, 1996).

Lindsey Napier is a lecturer in Social work at the University of Sydney. She came to academia after extensive practice experience, including front-line family welfare and public sector mental health work in London, local government and health service social work in Sydney and a long stint as social work adviser on health policy in the New South Wales state government. Her political work in the women's health and self-help movements and her research into the politics of reproduction have given way to researching and developing the new 'issue-based' curriculum for the final years of the social work degree. Central to this is the development of collaboration in teaching, writing and research with social workers in public health and welfare agencies. She holds academic and professional qualifications from Aberdeen, Edinburgh and Sydney universities and from the London School of Economics.

Bob Pease is a Senior Lecturer in the Department of Social Work at the Royal Melbourne Institute of Technology. He has written extensively on gender issues for men and is the author of *Men and Sexual Politics*. He has recently completed a PhD on profeminist men's politics and practices and is co-founder of Men Against Sexual Assault in Melbourne and founder of the White Ribbon Campaign against men's violence.

Isaac Prilleltensky is a fellow of the division of community psychology of the American Psychological Association. He is the author of *The Morals and Politics of Psychology: Psychological Discourse and the Status Quo* (SUNY Press, 1994), and co-editor of *Critical Psychology* (Sage, 1997) and of *Promoting Family Wellness and Preventing Child Maltreatment* (forthcoming).

Amy Rossiter is a Senior Lecturer at Atkinson College, the University of York, Ontario, Canada. She has published widely in the field of feminism, postmodernism and ethics.

Liz Trinder is a lecturer and researcher at the University of East Anglia. She has published widely on postmodern feminism and research in social work.

Richard Walsh-Bowers is Professor of Psychology at Wilfrid Laurier University, Waterloo, Ontario, Canada. He has contributed to the literature in community psychology, feminist psychology, and the history and ethics of psychology. He received his university's Outstanding Teacher Award of 1999. In his other lives, he is an actor and director in community and university theatre, and he was a candidate for the New Democratic Party in the 1999 Ontario provincial election.

Acknowledgements

The editors would like to thank all the contributors to this book and would particularly like to thank Pauline Brier from Bradford University, for her time and the excellent administrative support she provided.

Introduction

Jan Fook and Brid Featherstone

Can postmodern feminist understandings allow us as social workers to resist domination and if so, how? Is it either possible or desirable to unite postmodern thinking with 'movements' such as feminism which are concerned with political action? Or does postmodernism with its insistence that there is no possibility of 'innocent' knowledge undermine any basis for political change? Does the postmodern focus on difference inevitably hinder possibilities for solidarity? Does the questioning of identities and categories leave us without any tools to challenge oppression? What does it mean 'practically' to research/practise from a feminist postmodern perspective? The chapters presented in this book in varying ways engage with these difficult questions. Perspectives drawn from social theory, in particular postmodernism and feminism and postmodern feminism are applied to 'social work' which has itself to be viewed as a contested activity or set of activities.

The first two chapters provide the context for the subsequent discussions. Barbara Fawcett and Brid Featherstone in Chapter 1 focus on contemporary issues within feminism/s with regard to postmodernism and postmodernity and explore current debates about knowledge, subjectivity, difference and power. They interrogate some of the key political dilemmas facing the feminist engagement with postmodernism and highlight the work of a range of writers who are concerned with some, if not all of the above questions. In Chapter 2, Jan Fook and Amy Rossiter strike an 'optimistic' note arguing that postmodern feminism is a crisis for social work which has created important political openings. It has initiated a crisis of knowledge by raising questions about the authority and legitimacy of social work's claim to special knowledge. In addition, it has provoked a crisis of identity by casting doubt on social work's historical assumption of 'innocent' help. However, they argue that these two crises open up important spaces for a chastised social work which is better able to align with social justice.

The following two chapters are concerned with the 'doing' of research within social work. In Chapter 3 Liz Trinder critically reviews contemporary approaches to research in social work. She then moves on to consider the potential of poststructuralist and postmodern feminism, particularly in relation to the deconstructing of assumptions about 'innocent' research practices. She is particularly attracted to the emphasis in such perspectives on the deconstruction of fixed gender categories and she explores the consequent possibilities for 'change'. The chapter combines a discussion of epistemological and methodological questions with details of some of the components of a possible postmodern feminist approach to social work research practice. In Chapter 4, Barbara Fawcett concentrates on making connections between theory and research practice. She examines how perspectives drawn from postmodern feminism can be used to inform the research project she carried out in the United Kingdom on the meanings associated with disability. She explores how subjectivity is constructed and reconstructed in the discourse of participants. Some have a positive construct of disability which is an interesting addition to some of the assumptions which abound in the social work literature. She continues Trinder's emphasis on the desirability of avoiding fixed categories and argues that a sense of 'agency' can ensue from the acknowledgement and acceptance of changing subjectivities and social categories.

In the following section of the book, research into social work practice and issues relating to ethics and direct practice are highlighted. In Chapter 5, Rossiter, Prilleltensky and Walsh-Bowers, from a Canadian perspective, critically examine how practitioners in a number of settings understand and work with codes of ethics and understand 'ethical dilemmas'. They found that the practice of professional ethics is unlikely to involve the application of a universalist code. Rather, practitioners try to negotiate ethical decisions, within what they name as organisational 'tension sites' which are influenced by broader social forces (which are both economic and social). Rossiter *et al.* hence locate professional ethics within social relations and lament the focus within codes of ethics on the individual practitioner. They bring together, perhaps surprisingly, the analyses of Habermas and feminist postmodernists and they offer pointers towards radically rethinking the relations between larger social forces, organisations, individuals and ethics. Chapter 6 is concerned with the hoary old issues about theory/practice and expertise in social work. This chapter, from Australia, is based on research with a range of practitioners at differing stages of their professional careers. Jan Fook asks important questions in a current context (not solely applicable to Australia unfortunately) about how social workers can find meaning and direction when the contexts in which they work are changing and uncertain. Furthermore, in a situation of ongoing fragmentation of skills and organisational models of delivery, she asks how can a discourse of professional practice be developed which acknowledges situatedness, but at the same time provides the possibility of communicating meaningfully across diverse contexts.

The next section of the book focuses on practice issues such as mothers who physically abuse their children (Featherstone) and masculinity/masculinities (Pease). These chapters are based on research carried out by the authors and both explore the 'process' of researching. Brid Featherstone, from a perspective influenced by feminism, postmodernism and psychoanalysis reflects on her own research journey and the complexities involved in researching mothers' accounts. She argues that in qualitative research, which is concerned with 'sensitive' areas as much social work research inevitably is, considerable thought needs to be devoted to process. She highlights some of the process issues which became apparent in her face-to-face interviewing with mothers. She argues that a story-telling approach may hold out progressive possibilities for both interviewer and interviewee and is also more congruent with her leanings towards feminism, postmodernism and psychoanalysis. Bob Pease in Chapter 8 describes a number of research methods used in researching masculinity. He argues, in contrast to Trinder, that some standpoint perspectives are helpful and do not lead to essentialism. He is concerned to construct a profeminist men's standpoint in researching masculinity and considers this vital if men are to challenge their positions within patriarchy. He acknowledges his debt to postmodernism in its emphasis on the importance of moving away from fixed notions of subjectivity. He regards such a move away from essentialist positions as vital for the possibilities of change for and by men.

In Chapter 9, Lindsey Napier, in a reflective piece, explores how her thinking/teaching/practising in relation to death and dying have evolved over the years. She relates how she gradually lost faith with models of health care which promised certainty, based on assumptions that a clear knowledge of 'cause' will lead to foolproof methods of 'treatment'. She also notes how exclusionary categories of 'ordinary' and 'extraordinary' deaths are devised to aid professional practice. She argues that despite all the knowledge, personal, professional and academic, that she has at her disposal, certain knowledge about death and dying will always be out of reach. These are experiences which cannot be understood through social categorisation. Instead, she maintains that our best hope is to start engaging in dialogue, with a preparedness to listen, learn and reflect. Then it may be possible to give meaning to death and dying through engaging with the plurality of concrete and local understandings.

Finally, in Chapter 10, Vivienne Bozalek reflects on her experience as a white South African social work educator and she notes the paramountcy of issues of categorisation and difference in this arena. In a historical context which oppressively encoded racial difference, she questions the relevance of a form of postmodernism which irresponsibly valorises difference. She argues for a reconstructive postmodernism in which, in specific contexts, essentialised notions of ethnicity, race and gender are accepted in so far as they assist in discovering heritage and discursive positions. However, she additionally maintains that a broader transcendent vision which ultimately challenges these fixed categories is also necessary.

The authors who have contributed to this book come from Australia, Canada, South Africa and the United Kingdom. They clearly do not hold uniform theoretical perspectives, but all have been influenced by and engage with postmodern feminism. Accordingly, a key intention of the book is to challenge current thinking in the field of social work and to enable the reader to appraise the utility of orientations drawn from postmodern feminism for researching and practising in social work.

Chapter 1

Setting the scene

An appraisal of notions of postmodernism, postmodernity and postmodern feminism

Barbara Fawcett and Brid Featherstone

Introduction

Feminism has a contested and controversial history. Feminists have variously embraced liberal, Marxist and radical orientations and the influence of these diverse perspectives, together with the contribution made by Black feminisms, has been both dynamic and divisive. Within feminism(s), postmodernism has provoked wide-ranging reactions, ranging from the hostile, to the indifferent, to the creative. In relation to the latter, many feminist writers have directed their attention towards reframing postmodernist debates in ways which retain feminism's critical edge while rejecting notions of objectivity and all pervasive truth claims.

This introductory chapter will engage with current debates and will appraise conceptualisations that can, in various ways, be seen to be both postmodernist and feminist. In this context, the relationship between poststructural and postmodern perspectives will be examined. Some of the criticisms directed towards postmodernism will be explored and understandings of postmodernism reviewed. The utility of postmodernism for feminism will then be appraised by focusing on knowledge paradigms, understandings of subjectivity, conceptualisations of difference and considerations of power.

Poststructural and postmodern perspectives

The relationship between poststructural and postmodern perspectives is not clear cut and there are many differences of opinion as to whether they can be seen to relate to similar broad areas. Sarup, for example, asserts: 'In my opinion poststructuralists like Foucault, Derrida and Lyotard are postmodernists. There are so many similarities between post structuralist theories and postmodern practices that it is difficult to make a clear distinction between them' (1993: 144).

Huyssen (1990), however, disagrees and argues that poststructuralism is 'primarily a discourse of and about modernism'. He maintains: 'It is as if the creative powers of modernism had migrated into theory and come to full self-consciousness in the poststructuralist text' (Huyssen, 1990: 259–60). However, arguably, Huyssen bases this assertion on a particular reading of modernism and says:

> But if poststructuralism can be seen as the *revenant* of modernism in the guise of theory, then that would also be precisely what makes it postmodern. It is a postmodernism that works itself out not as a rejection of modernism, but rather as a retrospective reading which, in some cases is fully aware of modernism's limitations and failed political ambitions.
>
> (Huyssen, 1990: 261)

Butler   pertinently points to the different associations between poststructuralism and postmodernism which pertain in America and in France. She says that:

> On this side of the Atlantic [America] and in recent discourse, the terms 'postmodernism' or 'poststructuralism' settle the differences among those positions in a single stroke, providing a substantive, a noun, that includes those positions as so many of its modalities or permutations.
>
> (Butler, 1995: 36)

Butler prefers to talk about poststructuralism rather than postmodernism and goes on to say that in France in particular the two areas are very much in dispute.

Overall, it would appear that the debate continues. However, Barrett (1992) maintains that to explore the relationship between contemporary feminist and social theory it is necessary to cite postmodern as well as poststructural arguments. Accordingly, for the purposes of this chapter and for the book as a whole the term 'postmodern' will be used to refer to both poststructural and postmodern perspectives.

Feminism against postmodernism

In many respects feminism can be seen to have much in common with postmodernism. Both are concerned to challenge one of the defining characteristics of modernism, which is the projected universal validity of masculine context-specific knowledge claims. However, feminism has been historically and theoretically a modernist movement (Hekman, 1990: 2). Liberal and socialist feminisms, in particular, despite their differences, have both been rooted in the emancipatory impulses of modernism. Modern categories, such as those relating to equality and rights have provided women with the weapons to fight against their oppression. Lovibond (1989), for example, has argued that the rejection of modernist categories such as reason, equality, universal rights and emancipation will deprive women of important weapons. Furthermore, '[d]eriving norms and concepts of justice from local and particular domains is problematical ... since it is often local domains – like the family, office or conservative neighbourhoods or towns – that oppress women and negate their rights' (Lovibond, 1989, in Best and Kellner, 1991: 209–10).

Brodrib (1992) is dismissive of poststructural and postmodern orientations, preferring to concentrate on the politics of reproduction. She maintains that as it is only white men who have historically been recognised as subjects, it is somewhat suspect for this notion to be abolished, just as white women and black people are also asserting their rights to be subjects. Christian (1988) and Hartsock (1990) question postmodern[1] critiques of humanism and structuralism, particularly with regard to the relativistic implications for Third World and minority cultures in terms of their efforts to gain legitimacy for their struggles.

Benhabib (1995) makes links between the key theses of the postmodern position as outlined by Flax (1990) and feminism. She distinguishes between 'strong' analyses, which according to Benhabib are incompatible with the feminist project and 'weak' analyses, which she regards as being similar to feminist critiques. Accordingly, it is only these latter critiques which can be utilised. Benhabib maintains:

Postmodernism can teach us the theoretical and political traps of why utopias and foundational thinking can go wrong, but it should not lead to a retreat from utopia altogether. For we, as women, have much to lose by giving up the utopian hope in the wholly other.

(1995: 30)

The question of postmodernism

The question of postmodernism is surely a question, for is there, after all, something called postmodernism? Is it an historical characterisation, a certain kind of theoretical position, and what does it mean for a term that has described a certain aesthetic practice now to apply to social theory and to feminist social and political theory in particular?

(Butler, 1995: 35)

Numerous writers have become involved with exploring what postmodernism 'is' and how 'it' relates to postmodernity. It is not the intention to rehearse the debates in any detail here. However, it is important in terms of contemporary debates, to note that postmodernism is itself a contested term and needs deconstructing. It is not helpful either from a positive or oppositional stance to assume its coherence and there can be seen to be important political implications. Before exploring these it is worth noting that in this chapter a distinction is made between postmodernity and postmodernism. Accordingly, postmodernity is seen to refer to a broad set of changes which characterise contemporary Western societies and postmodernism to particular theoretical positions. It is accepted that such a distinction is contested.

Theorists differ as to whether postmodernity is a new condition or a continuation of changes intrinsic to modernity. Bauman (1992) regards postmodernity as a new condition, but one which is relational in that it involves modernity facing up to itself. Bauman sees postmodernity as relating to a new type of society characterised by a rejection of universal standards of beauty or truth. The ethical paradox of this condition is that the fullness of moral choice is restored to agents at the same time as they are deprived of the comfort of the universal guidance that modern self-confidence promised. Consumer conduct moves into the position occupied by labour and individuals are engaged morally by society and functionally by the social system as consumers rather than as producers. With consumption firmly established as the focus and the playground for individual freedom, the future of capitalism looks more secure than ever. Social control becomes easier and less costly as expensive methods of control are disposed of or replaced by more efficient methods of seduction. The capitalist system in this phase does not need, or needs only marginally, traditional mechanisms of securing its reproduction, such as consensus-aimed political legitimation. Culture has lost its relevance to the survival and perpetuation of the system or rather it contributes to such survival through its heterogeneity and fissiparousness rather than the levelling impact of civilising crusades. The market thrives on variety and has proved to be the arch-enemy of uniformity. Despite writing of systems and structures, Bauman (1995) argues that we need to move away from the notion of the social world as a cohesive totality with neatly arranged hierarchies of power, towards visions of a fluid, changeable social setting.

It is important to acknowledge that there are considerable debates about the legitimacy of views which argue that postmodernity is new. Clarke (1996) argues that engaging with terms such as postmodernity or postmodernism runs the risk of historical amnesia in that it encourages a failure to look at continuities and to recognise how changes today merely represent forms of restructuring class relations in the pursuit of profit accumulation. Others such as Giddens (1984, 1991) argue that modernity has not yet run its course and that we are now in late modernity. While these debates are important, perhaps a useful operating strategy is not to get too caught up with labels, but rather to use whatever analyses appear helpful in order to understand what is going on. Consequently, although this book locates itself within postmodernism it is apparent that various authors use a range of theorists from a range of backgrounds to illuminate the issues with which they grapple. This, it can be argued is particularly characteristic of the ways in which many feminists engage with social theory.

It is important to recognise that those who engage with postmodernism may be doing so with quite different political agendas. This is clearly relevant when considering feminist involvement with postmodernism. However, a range of feminist writers are engaging critically with postmodern ideas in order to understand and challenge, as well as develop the means to fight injustice and oppression. In order to focus the discussion the following areas will be explored: knowledge production, subjectivity, difference and power.

Feminism for postmodernism

Producing useful knowledge

Harding (1991) conceptualises feminist contributions to the social sciences in the following ways: feminist empiricism, standpoint feminism and postmodernism. She argues that feminist empiricism is concerned to rectify the male bias of faulty science. It points out that what has passed for science is in fact the world as perceived by men, what appears to be objectivity is really sexism, and the types of questions which have traditionally been asked have excluded women and their interests and needs (Smart, 1992: 77–8). It does not challenge established traditions about methodology and epistemology but concentrates on filling in the gaps in mainstream science.

It is standpoint feminism which has arguably become most dominant in the feminist research literature and in particular in the literature used within social work in the United Kingdom, particularly in work concerning sexual violence and abuse (see Kelly, 1992).

> This ... approach originates in Hegel's insight into the rela-
> tionship between the master and the slave and the development
> of Hegel's perception into the 'proletarian standpoint' by Marx,
> Engels and George Lukács. The assertion is that human activity
> or 'material life', not only structures but sets limits on human
> understanding: what we do shapes and constrains what we can
> know.
>
> (Harding, 1991: 120)

Feminist standpoint theorists believe that the standpoint of women and feminism is less partial and distorted than the picture which emerges from conventional research. The grounds for this claim lie, according to Harding, in the distinctiveness of women's material and emotional lives. She argues in more recent work that in limited but important respects social disadvantage creates a limited but important epistemic advantage. She also argues that socially located knowledge can be universally valid.

In recent years debates have emerged about the role of 'experience' in relation to standpoint feminism and in the United States particularly, the critiques of women of colour, as well as the growing influence of postmodernism, have meant that there can appear to be a convergence between theorists who have appeared more opposed in the past. For example, in relation to 'experience', Harding has argued that some thinkers assume that standpoint theories must be grounded in women's experiences. However, she argues that women's experiences in themselves or the things women say cannot provide reliable grounds for knowledge claims about nature and social relations:

> After all, experience itself is shaped by social relations: for example, women have had to *learn* to define as rape those sexual assaults that occur within marriage. Women had experienced those assaults not as something which could be called rape, but only as part of the range of heterosexual sex that wives could expect.
>
> (Harding, 1991: 123)

There is a convergence here to a limited extent with the views of Jana Sawicki (1991) who has become associated with postmodern/poststructural perspectives. Sawicki writes that:

> Narratives of oppressed groups are important insofar as they empower these groups by giving them a voice in the struggle over interpretations without claiming to be epistemically privileged or incontestable. They are not denied the 'authority' of experience if, by 'authority,' one means the power to introduce that experience as a basis for analysis, and thereby to create new self-understandings. What is denied is the authority of unanalyzed experience.
>
> (1991: 169)

Both writers distance themselves from perspectives which see 'experience' as unproblematic. Sawicki identifies strongly, however, with a theme of postmodernism which will be detailed more fully later and which sees feminist knowledge itself as problematic. Harding, in contrast, whilst acknowledging the limitations of feminist knowledge does appear to see it as ultimately unproblematic.

As Hekman (1996) has noted, Hartsock (1996) a leading standpoint theorist, increasingly writes not of *the* feminist standpoint that defines the oppression of women, but of situated knowledges. These are 'a plural conception of the truth and knowledge that allows for multiple realities' (Hekman, 1996: 5). This is a shift which can be seen to be influenced by the critiques of women of colour, as well as by the challenge of postmodernism. Hartsock's (1996) work in particular, is marked by awareness of the importance of oppression as a result of 'race' and 'imperialism'. Her argument is that despite dangers such as co-option 'at the level of epistemology there are a number of similarities that can provide the basis for differing groups to understand each other and form alliances' (ibid.: 52). This she poses as an alternative to the dead-end oppositions of postmodernism which she sees as rejecting the possibility of knowledge altogether. However, it appears that she makes common cause with other feminist postmodernists when she argues, with regard to situated knowledges, that rather 'than accept(ing) the false challenge of omnipotence or impotence, these knowledges can be recognized as limited and changing, as ongoing achievements of continuing struggles' (1996: 52). This can be seen to have some congruence with the calls of Fraser and Nicholson (1993) for 'a post-modernist, pragmatic, fallibilistic mode of feminist theorising that would retain social–critical emancipatory force ' (Fraser, 1995: 62).

However, there appear to be important differences between standpoint theorists and postmodern feminists which have relevance for practice. The most important concerns what might be characterised as a sense of faith or hope about the status of feminist knowledge itself. While standpoint theorists such as Hartsock (1996) do recognise that feminist knowledge might be limited and limiting, she does, in a similar way to Harding (1991), seem to see it as ultimately emancipatory. Flax (1992a), a feminist who engages with postmodernism and psychoanalysis, by contrast, expresses strong reservations about this. She argues that standpoint theorists like other feminist theorists are dreaming both of the impossible and the undesirable in their attempts to find what she calls 'innocent knowledge'. The desire for innocent knowledge, arises, she argues, from a wish for some sort of truth which will tell us how to act in the world in ways which benefit all. For her, one of the fundamental antinomies of Enlightenment thinking shared by feminists is that of superstition/domination versus knowledge /freedom (emancipation). The assumption here is that domination and emancipation are a binary pair and displacing one inevitably creates space for the other (Flax, 1992a: 457). In arguing the above, Flax is drawing to some extent on the work of Foucault who argued that oppositional discourses often extend the very relations of domination that they are resisting (Foucault, in Rabinow, 1984).

However, feminists who align with postmodernism are critical of many postmodern writings with regard to knowledge production. While accepting postmodern critiques of universalist theorising and subsequently rejecting, for example, any attempts to develop one theory which explains the position of women worldwide or the original cause of women's oppression, there is a clear concern by postmodern feminists to retain some form of large-scale theorising in order to understand the systematicity as well as the diversity of women's oppression. Fraser and Nicholson (1993) have consistently asserted that large historical narratives are not inconsistent with postmodern theory. Both large- and small-scale narratives are required as one will counteract the distorting tendencies of the other. Local genealogising narratives counteract the tendency of large-scale accounts to congeal into 'quasi meta-narratives, while larger contextualising accounts help to prevent local narratives from devolving into simple demonstrations of difference' (Fraser, 1995: 62).

Fraser and Nicholson (1993) do make common cause with postmodernists such as Lyotard when they argue that such theorising does not require grounding in the sense of the God's eye view of foundationalist thought, but they make it clear that this does not mean abolishing all criteria for evaluating knowledge. Fraser (1995) asserts: 'we might posit a relation to history that is at once antifoundationalist and politically engaged, while promoting a field of multiple historiographies that is both contextualised and provisionally totalizing' (1995: 71–2).

Subjectivity

An important aim of much feminism could be said to be related to changing societal structures so that women become subjects of history. However, by opening up spaces for women to tell the stories that have been suppressed by men in their theorising about the world (stories about maternal practices, for example), they have challenged what it means to be a subject. Attention to the everyday and to neglected areas (such as what kind of thinking does mothering require) obliges a reconsideration of what being a subject involves. Much Enlightenment thought seems to see subjects as disembodied, unlocated individuals. Feminist thinking, in contrast, has stressed the importance of interdependence and location in the construction of subjectivity and has illustrated how such aspects are suppressed by men and by dominant notions of subjectivity.

There are a number of tensions here for feminists who engage with postmodernism. A common critique from other feminists, as highlighted earlier, is that postmodernism abandons the subject just when white women and people of colour are asserting their right to be subjects or re-defining what it means to be a subject. This is not purely of theoretical significance, but has important political implications. Furthermore, the focus by some theorists on the role of language in the construction of subjects is seen as problematic. Writers who argue that the subject is an effect of discourses or those who speak of the subject as a position in language are critiqued by feminists such as Benhabib (1995). She argues that the subject viewed as another position in language, can no longer 'master' and create the distance between itself and the chain of significations in which it is immersed, in order to reflect upon and creatively alter them. Consequently, important political questions are raised here about the possibility of women having agency.

According to feminist postmodernists such as Hekman (1990, 1995), however, there are a range of postmodern positions on the question of the subject. One is concerned with destabilising the subject through an emphasis on fiction, play and fantasy. She argues that this strand tends towards nihilism and political passivity. However, there is another strand which is concerned with redefining the subject of the Marxist tradition and articulating a resistant and discursively constituted subject and it is here that she appears to locate herself.

Most feminist postmodernists are concerned, to varying degrees, with continuing a project of resistance to oppression. However, they do differ on the role of the subject in relation to this project. Butler (1995) urges us to bid farewell to the 'doer' behind the deed and to the self as the subject of a life narrative. Flax (1992a) in contrast, while acknowledging the constructed nature of the subject and cautioning against attempts to discover authenticity or the 'truth', argues that we do have a 'core self' which is developed relationally and which is very important in terms of fostering subjects who can recognise each other and co-operate together. This 'core self', she stresses, differs from the unitary self of Enlightenment thought which assumes that independence, coherence and rationality are desirable and possible attributes. It is a self which is formed through relationships, crucially those with early care-givers and recognises interdependence and the ability to be 'different' in different contexts. However, it is also a sense of self which retains throughout, the ability to construct narratives of the 'self' with a sense of past, present and future.

Difference

Questions of difference have been a central concern for feminists for some time. Difference has been used to refer to differences between women, as well as to differences between women and men. The question of difference has also been central for many postmodern writers. In particular, the construction of differences as well as the political implications have been addressed. As Haber (1994) notes, Lyotard, among others has argued that a key problem with what he called grand narratives, such as Marxism, is that they have tended to homogenise and close off differences. Techniques such as genealogy and deconstruction allow for the hearing of marginalised voices and exploring how particular concerns are silenced in political struggles. Haber (1994) notes, however, that there is often a problem with male postmodernist writers in that they universalise difference and equate all unity with terror. Such formulations can be seen to disallow the identity formations which are necessary for political resistance.

In terms of differences between men and women, postmodern feminists have been concerned to move beyond characteristic and important second-wave feminist positions. These are that such differences are socially constructed or that (and this is a more contested feminist position associated with cultural feminism (Eisenstein, 1984)), that women's difference from men can be valorised. In relation to this area, Flax (1992b), from a different position, writes not of men and women, but of gender relations arguing that a relational understanding treats the notion of difference itself as problematic and allows us to explore how differences are reproduced and maintained in ongoing psychic and material practices. Hollway (1989) also provides a vivid illustration of this in her exploration of how men and women position themselves in relation to each other and with regard to the discourses available to them.

In terms of differences between women, 'race' at certain periods, particularly in the United Kingdom and the United States, has featured significantly, although differences relating to class, age, sexuality and disability have also been emphasised. There can be seen to be a number of important points of convergence and divergence between postmodern feminists and those who resist the label. As already demonstrated, Harding (1991) and Hartsock (1996) acknowledge the implications, particularly of 'race', for knowledge production. Points of divergence with postmodern feminists have already been indicated and relate to the concern that even if it were possible to produce an all inclusive theory, that is one which registers all the indices of oppression in women's lives, it would also generate, as postmodern feminists such as Flax (1992a) argue, its own regulatory impulses.

However, most postmodern feminists firmly eschew a tendency in male writings to valorise or celebrate difference for its own sake. This is in line with a concern to explore why some differences lead to domination and to make difference a resource *for* rather than an obstacle *against* political change (Sawicki, 1991). Williams (1996), for example, has tried to integrate postmodern considerations of difference with feminist concerns about difference and the feminist project of challenging unequal power relations. She deconstructs difference by associating terms such as diversity, difference and division with particular political possibilities and challenges. By diversity, she refers to difference viewed as a shared collective experience; one which is not necessarily associated with subordination and inequality. An example here could be a shared language. Difference relates to a situation where a shared collective experience/identity (around or combining gender and sexuality, for example), forms the basis for resistance against the positioning of that identity as subordinate. By division she refers to the translation of a shared experience into a form of domination and an example here could be being a white man in a particular context. She stresses that these are not fixed categories. This analysis can be seen to suggest that none of the categories need to be automatically viewed as reactionary or emancipatory, although the associated political possibilities are variously circumscribed. This discussion opens up questions around whether expressing difference inevitably leads to a form of closure which prevents groups moving beyond their own interests to recognise commonalities with others.

An inter-related concern focuses on the relationship between subjectivity and difference. 'Individuals' can be located within a range of complex and contradictory categories, for example, those of white, disabled, middle-class woman and follow a 'life trajectory' within time and space. As many social theorists, including those who refuse the label postmodern have pointed out, the possibility of constructing one's life and of re-fashioning oneself is arguably a central motif of contemporary Western culture (see for example Giddens, 1992). Furthermore, the projects of others whom we build lives with, may or may not converge and disrupt our location within categories. A common example is that of a woman whose partner leaves her leading to downward class mobility. Areas such as mothering and 'disability', viewed as experience and as process, also involve the negotiation of shifting identities across time and space.

Power

For those concerned with challenging injustice, exploring and understanding power relations are central activities. This has proved, arguably, *the* area where feminists have disagreed, with regard to the utility or otherwise of postmodern insights. With regard to explorations of power, the work of Foucault has undoubtedly been influential. As with many writers, whose work spans a number of decades, his writings can and have been read in a number of different ways. In particular, his later work on ethics has prompted considerable debate and has lent credence to a view that it is not appropriate to locate him within postmodernism (a location he himself contested). However, arguably, any discussion of postmodernism and power has to take account of his work and a brief résumé is given below.

With regard to conceptualisations of power, Foucault moves away from an absolutist, repressive view of power and presents a perspective which regards power as productive. He argues that power is relational and that it is exercised rather than possessed, emanating from the 'bottom up' in routine social practices. He makes what can be seen as a crucial distinction between power and domination, maintaining that power relations enable and produce rather than merely prohibit. Accordingly, although situations of domination leave little room for resistance, power relations, according to Foucault, always contain the possibility of resistance. Similarly, as power is not located in one place, power relations and points of resistance are always multiple.

In his earlier works, Foucault tended to call his approach archaeology (Foucault, 1972; Merquior, 1985). In his later writings, he developed a form of critical enquiry which he called a genealogy of modern power (Foucault, 1980, 1981b). The main focus of genealogy is to understand the conditions which make certain social practices or 'regimes of practices' (Foucault, 1981b: 5) acceptable at a particular moment in time. Foucault by the use of the genealogy of power focused on how power was exercised through the interplay of discourses (McNeil, 1993). As Cain (1993) points out, it was by using this method that led Foucault to claim that the exercise of power creates knowledge, while knowledge produces the effects of power. His use of genealogy, in terms of the operation of power and knowledge, as Ramazanoglu (1993) asserts, had wide-ranging implications for concepts of emancipation and oppression. Rather than focusing on emancipation from oppression, Foucault indicated that emphasis ought to be placed on producing alternative discourses, alternative forms of power and alternative forms of the 'self' as a means of changing political relations.

Foucault's work has been variously received by feminists who have engaged with postmodern orientations. Ramazanoglu and Holland (1993) for example, accept the significance of Foucault's work, but call for a 'middle ground' position on power. They are particularly concerned that his perspective moves away from oppressor/oppressed dualisms and they draw attention to the tension between his view that power is everywhere and ever present and his references to particular concentrations of power. However, Diamond and Quinby (1988), Flax (1990), Sawicki (1991) and Faith (1994) among others, emphasise the importance and utility of Foucault's exploration of power/knowledge regimes for social criticism and feminism. Sawicki (1991) and Faith (1994) for example, critically flag up radical elements which highlight the fact that resistance and struggle should be examined as the key to understanding and dismantling subordination and that, like power, resistance is heterogeneous, plural and diverse in form. They also pick up on Foucault's assertions that where there is power there is always resistance, with resistance being viewed as an integral part of power in that it is an element of its functioning as well as a source of its perpetual disorder (Foucault, 1983).

Overall, in relation to postmodern feminism, although Foucault paid little attention to gender divisions, his work has undoubtedly generated ideas and has also lent itself to creative development. In particular, his emphasis on power as productive and upon power relations operating at the micro level, has opened up further areas for analysis. However, it is Foucault's conceptualisation that power's relationship to knowledge is never separable because within each society there is a regime of truth with its own particular mechanisms for producing truth (Diamond and Quinby 1988: x), that can be seen to have provided a particular 'catalyst' for postmodern feminism.

Conclusion

The intention in this introductory chapter has been to provide an overview of the concepts and the arguments, to place the debates in context and to provide the backdrop for the discussions which will take place throughout this book. It has also to be re-emphasised that none of the contributors are arguing for a non-critical acceptance of perspectives drawn from postmodern feminism, rather, the concern is to foster dialogue and to promote the engagement and application of the ideas to researching and practising in social work.

Note

1 Cain (1993) and Hartsock (1990) refer to poststructural perspectives. However, as outlined in this chapter, for the purposes of this book, poststructuralist and postmodern orientations are being conflated.

Bibliography

Barrett, M. (1992) 'Words and things: materialism and method in contemporary feminist analysis', in M. Barrett and A. Phillips (eds) *Destabilising Theory: Contemporary Feminist Debates*, Cambridge: Polity Press.

Bauman, Z. (1995) *Life in Fragments: Essays in Postmodern Morality,* Oxford: Blackwell.

Benhabib, S. (1992) *Situating the Self. Gender, Community and Postmodernism in Contemporary Ethics*, London: Routledge.

—— (1995) 'Feminism and postmodernism', in L. Nicholson (ed.) *Feminist Contentions: A Philosophical Exchange*, London: Routledge.

Best, S. and Kellner, D. (1991) *Postmodern Theory: Critical Interrogations*, Basingstoke: Macmillan.

Brodrib, S. (1992) *Nothing Mat(t)ers: A Feminist Critique of Postmodernism*, Melbourne: Spinnifex.

Butler, J. (1995) 'Contingent foundations', in L. Nicholson (ed.) *Feminist Contentions: A Philosophical Exchange*, London: Routledge.

Cain, M. (1993) 'Foucault, feminism and feeling: what Foucault can and cannot contribute to feminist epistemology', in C. Ramazanoglu (ed.) *Up Against Foucault: Explorations of Some Tensions Between Foucault and Feminism*, London: Routledge.

Christian, B. (1988) 'The race for theory', *Feminist Studies* 14: 67–9.

Clarke, J. (1996) 'After social work', in N. Parton (ed.) *Social Theory, Social Change and Social Work*, London: Routledge.

Derrida, J. (1978) *Writing and Difference*, trans. A. Bass, Chicago: University of Chicago Press.

Di Stefano, C. (1990) 'Dilemmas of difference', in L. Nicholson (ed.) *Feminism/Postmodernism*, London: Routledge.

Diamond, I. and Quinby, L. (1988) (eds) *Feminism and Foucault*, Boston: Northeastern University Press.

Dreyfus, H.L. and Rabinow, P. (eds) (1993) *Michel Foucault: Beyond Structuralism and Hermeneutics*, Chicago: University of Chicago Press.

Eisenstein, H. (1984) *Contemporary Feminist Thought*, London: Allen and Unwin.

Faith, K. (1994) 'Resistance: lessons from Foucault and feminism', in H.L. Radtke and H.J. Stam (eds) *Power/Gender Social Relations in Theory and Practice*, London: Sage.

Fawcett, B. (1998) 'Disability and social work: applications from poststructuralism, postmodernism and feminism', *British Journal of Social Work* 28: 263–77.

Fawcett, B. and Featherstone, B. (1998) 'Quality assurance and evaluation in social work in a postmodern era', in J. Carter (ed.) *Postmodernity and the Fragmentation of Welfare*, London: Routledge.

Flax, J. (1990) *Thinking Fragments, Psychoanalysis, Feminism and Postmodernism in the Contemporary West*, Berkeley, CA: University of California Press.

—— (1992a) 'The end of innocence', in J. Butler and J. Scott (eds) *Feminists Theorise the Political*, London: Routledge.

—— (1992b) 'Beyond equality, gender, justice and difference', in L. Bock and S. James (eds) *Beyond Equality and Difference*, London: Routledge.

Foucault, M. (1972) *The Archaeology of Knowledge*, London: Tavistock.

—— (1979) *Discipline and Punish*, Harmondsworth: Penguin.

—— (1980) *Michel Foucault: Power/Knowledge: Selected Interviews and Other Writings 1972–1977*, ed. C. Gordon, Hemel Hempstead: Harvester Wheatsheaf.

—— (1981a) *The History of Sexuality, Volume One, An Introduction*, Harmondsworth: Pelican.

—— (1981b) 'Question of method: an interview with Michel Foucault', *Ideology and Consciousness* 8: 1–14.

—— (1983) *Michel Foucault: Beyond Structuralism and Hermeneutics*, eds H.L. Drefus and P. Rabinow, Chicago: University of Chicago Press.

—— (1986) *The History of Sexuality, Volume Two, The Use of Pleasure*, Harmondsworth: Viking.

—— (1991) *The Foucault Reader*, ed. P. Rabinow, Harmondsworth: Penguin.

Fraser, N. (1995) 'False antithesis', in L. Nicholson (ed.) *Feminist Contentions: A Philosophical Exchange*, London: Routledge.

Fraser, N. and Nicholson, L. (1993) 'Social criticism without philosophy: an encounter between feminism and postmodernism', in M. Docherty (ed.) *Postmodernism: A Reader*, Hemel Hempstead: Harvester Wheatsheaf.

Giddens, A. (1984) *The Constitution of Society*, Cambridge: Polity Press.

—— (1990) *The Consequences of Modernity*, Cambridge: Polity Press.

—— (1991) *Modernity and Self Identity*, Cambridge: Polity Press.

—— (1992) *The Transformation of Intimacy*, Cambridge: Polity Press.

Haber, H.F. (1994) *Beyond Post-modern Politics*, London: Routledge.

Habermas, J. (1981) 'Modernity versus postmodernity', *New German Critique* 22: 3–14.

Harding, S. (1986) *The Science in Question*, Ithaca, New York: Cornell University Press.

—— (1990) 'Feminism, science and the anti-enlightenment critique', in L. Nicholson (ed.) *Feminism/Postmodernism*, London: Routledge.

—— (1991) *Whose Science? Whose Knowledge? Thinking from Women's Lives*, Milton Keynes: Open University Press.

Hartsock, N. (1990) 'Foucault on power: a theory for women', in J. Nicholson (ed.) *Feminism/Postmodernism*, London: Routledge.

—— (1996) 'Postmodernism and political change: issues for feminist theory', in S. Hekman (ed.) *Feminist Interpretations of Michel Foucault*, Pennsylvania: Pennsylvania State University Press.

Hekman, S. (1990) *Gender and Knowledge: Elements of a Postmodern Feminism*, Cambridge: Polity Press.

—— (1995) *Moral Voices, Moral Selves: Carol Gilligan and Feminist Moral Theory*, Cambridge: Polity Press.

—— (ed.) (1996) *Feminist Interpretations of Foucault*, Pennsylvania: Pennsylvania State University Press.

Hollway, W. (1984) 'Gender, difference and the production of subjectivity', in J. Henriques, W. Hollway, C. Urwin, C, Venn and V.

Walkerdine (eds) *Changing the Subject: Psychology, Social Regulation and Subjectivity*, London: Methuen.

—— (1989) *Subjectivity and Method in Psychology: Gender, Meaning and Science*, London: Sage.

—— (1996) 'Gender and power in organizations', in B. Fawcett, B. Featherstone, J. Hearn and C. Toft (eds) *Violence and Gender Relations: Theories and Interventions*, London: Sage.

Huyssen, A. (1990) 'Mapping the postmodern', in L. Nicholson (ed.) *Feminism/Postmodernism*, London: Routledge.

Kelly, L. (1992) 'Journeying in reverse: possibilities and problems in feminist research on sexual violence', in L. Gelsthorpe and A. Morris (eds) *Feminist Perspectives in Criminology*, Milton Keynes: Open University Press.

Lovibond, S. (1989) 'Feminism and postmodernism', *New Left Review* 178: 5–28.

Lyotard, J.F. (1988) *The Differend: Phases in Dispute*, Manchester: Manchester University Press.

—— (1994) *The Postmodern Condition: A Report on Knowledge*, Manchester: Manchester University Press (originally published 1984).

Macdonell, D. (1986) *Theories of Discourse: An Introduction*, Oxford: Blackwell.

McNay, L. (1992) *Foucault and Feminism*, Oxford: Blackwell.

McNeil, M. (1993) 'Dancing with Foucault', in C. Ramazanoglu (ed.) *Up Against Foucault: Exploration of Some Tensions Between Foucault and Feminism*, London: Routledge.

Merquior, J.G. (1985) *Foucault,* London: Collins.

Moore, H.L. (1994) *A Passion for Difference*, Cambridge: Polity Press.

Nicholson, L. (1990) (ed.) *Feminism/Postmodernism*, London: Routledge.

—— (1995) *Feminist Contentions*, London: Routledge.

Rabinow, P. (ed.) (1984) *The Foucault Reader*, Harmondsworth: Penguin.

Ramazanoglu, C. (1993) (ed.) *Up Against Foucault: Explorations of Some Tensions Between Foucault and Feminism*, London: Routledge.

Ramazanoglu, C. and Holland, J. (1993) 'Women's sexuality and men's appropriation of desire', in C. Ramazanoglu (ed.) *Up Against Foucault*, London: Routledge.

Sarup, M. (1993) *Poststructuralism and Postmodernism*, Hemel Hempstead: Harvester Wheatsheaf.

Saussure, F. de (1974) *Course in General Linguistics*, London: Collins (original 1916).

Sawicki, J. (1991) *Disciplining Foucault: Feminism, Power and the Body*, London: Routledge.

Scott, J.W. (1994) 'Deconstructing equality-versus-difference: or the uses of poststructuralist theory for feminism', in L. McDowell and R. Pringle (eds) *Defining Women: Social Institutions and Gender Divisions*, Cambridge: Polity Press/Open University Press.

Segal, L. (1987) *Is the Future Female? Troubled Thoughts on Contemporary Feminism*, London: Virago.

Seidman, S. (1994) (ed.) *The Postmodern Turn: New Perspectives on Social Theory*, Cambridge: Cambridge University Press.

Smart, B. (1992) *Postmodernity*, London: Routledge.

Smart, C. (1992) 'Feminist approaches to criminology or postmodern woman meets atavistic man', in L. Gelsthorpe and A. Morris (eds) *Feminist Perspectives in Criminology*, Buckingham: Open University Press.

Weedon, C. (1987) *Feminist Practice and Poststructuralist Theory*, Oxford: Blackwell.

Williams, F. (1996) 'Postmodernism, feminism and the question of difference', in N. Parton (ed.) *Social Theory, Social Change and Social Work*, London: Routledge.

Chapter 2

The postmodern feminist condition

New conditions for social work

Amy Rossiter

Following from the overview of postmodern feminism in the previous chapter, this chapter explores the connections between postmodern feminism and the objectives of critical social work. It is clear that feminism grounds itself in a political struggle which aims at changing gender relations (Flax, 1990b). It is also clear that progressive social work shares a great deal of the political intentions of feminism (Sands and Nuccio, 1992) in that it requires emancipatory practices in its involvement with oppressed and marginalised people. However, in view of the criticism of postmodernism's failure to specify political grounds for action (Wapner, 1989), this chapter will examine postmodern feminism as a crisis for social work that has created important political openings. The work of the contributors of this book elaborates how those openings can be taken up in social work theory, practice and research.

In our view, postmodern feminism has undermined the conventional rationality of social work at two basic levels. It has initiated a crisis of knowledge, raising such questions as 'how do we know what we know?' and 'what authorises social work's claim to special knowledge?' It has also produced a crisis of identity as the postmodern critique casts doubts on social work's historical assumption about the innocence of providing help. These two overlapping crises open up important spaces for a chastised social work which is better able to align with social justice.

The crisis of knowledge

Those of us who undertook conventional social work education had few questions about the nature of reality. Social work theory is an outgrowth of an Enlightenment inheritance: it calls on totalising 'truths' which seek to provide unitary explanations of human nature. These explanations provide rough normative expectations for people, and those who fall outside these expectations, either by individual flaw, or the impress of bad social conditions become targets of social work intervention. In short, models and theories work to supply a description of reality from which social workers can organise practical intervention. Such descriptions have been legitimated under the aegis of science and scientific method. The adoption of the knowledge claims of science in social work has guaranteed 'truthful' descriptions of reality, thus legitimating the expertise on which social work's status as a profession arises.

The crisis for these conventions has derived from postmodernism's insistence that reality is an effect of language. The shift that has rocked modernity, and with it, social work, is the objection to modernism's conception of language as a transparent medium which grants humans access to unmediated reality. This shift began with the work of de Sassure (Henriques et al., 1984) who rejected the assumption that there is any necessary correspondence between a word as a sound, and the reality that is referenced by the word. This work opened the way for radical rethinking about relations between language, knowledge and power. In short, we have no innocent access to reality: reality is an effect of language because we cannot know outside of language. And language is social – made by humans. The very fact that language is social means that descriptions of reality are inevitably produced within the power relations of human society. We can have no brute reality – only the stories we tell about it. This shift immediately carries away the conventions of social work which rely on innocent descriptions of reality, and instantiates questions which take social work to the heart of power: who makes up social work realities? What are the interests? Who benefits? What are the limits of this knowledge?

What are the implications of the notion that 'All that we can know is what we say about the world – our talk, our sentences, our discourse, our texts' (C. Hawthorne quoted in Spivak, 1990: 17)? This notion is entirely incompatible with Enlightenment traditions which have sought to provide increasingly better notions about the foundations of human nature and human conduct. Such foundations are the origins of social work knowledge: for example, Freud's attempt to describe the human psyche, or Marx's understanding of the material base as the foundation of human conduct. Postmodernism ends the possibility of faith in foundations, leaving us with what Gayatri Spivak understands as 'a radical acceptance of vulnerability':

> The 'grands récits' are great narratives and the narrative has an end in view. It is a programme which tells how social justice is to be achieved. And I think the post-structuralists, if I understand them right, imagine again and again that when a narrative is constructed, something is left out. When an end is defined, other ends are rejected, and one might not know what those ends are. So I think what they are about is asking over and over again, what is left out.
>
> (Spivak, 1990: 18)

It is here that we can begin to understand the political project of postmodernism that feminism has taken up, and which it shares with social work. The idea that foundations, or 'grand récits' are but stories that are heard among stories that are not heard, prompts the refusal to privilege such foundations, thereby creating space for contesting marginality. When it is understood that a foundation is only a partial perspective, it also becomes clear that the representation of reality it adopts is produced in and through the location of the knower. Representations that get heard are empowered narratives. Indeed, rich avenues for feminist postmodern scholarship concern questions of power and representation. How have versions of the feminine been created through relations of power? In this sense, postmodernism, far from being the apolitical purveyor of relativism (Dews, 1989), signals a profound democratisation made possible through contesting representations by requiring accountability about who and what has been left out of the story. Peter Leonard signals this democratisation of knowledge when he says:

> The rules of exclusion that have operated so powerfully in social work to privilege forms and sources of knowledge that are eurocentric, patriarchal, and bourgeois are an essential means of ideological domination. The task of critical social work practice and education might be seen as the search for alternative sources of knowledge, both those that have been subordinated as part of the social mechanisms of class, gender and ethnic domination, and those that have flourished outside the discourses of objective scientific knowledge, in literature, myth and folklore.
>
> (Leonard, 1994: 22)

The implications for social work of the political project of questioning representations has created equally rich sites of investigation. Here, clients' perspectives have taken on a new importance. Seen as subjugated knowledge, the question of representation has allowed social work to decentre models and theories (Fook, Chapter 6) and instead install the client as an important site of knowledge. The focus of attention becomes clients' narratives (Gorman, 1993) and clients' ways of making meaning, rather than techniques for getting theories to work. Such a shift challenges an authoritarian professionalism by conceiving of help as that which emerges from the negotiation of two authentic stories – that of the client and the worker. It confronts social work with profound ethical questions about the contradictions between professionalism and commitment to social equality (Leonard, 1997).

Investigations of the construction of representation in social policy enables crucial critiques with clear political goals. For example, Nancy Fraser and Linda Gordon (1994) trace the powerful effect of notions of 'dependency' in American conceptions of welfare. They argue that dependence is associated with feminine weakness and that welfare policies that rely on notions of dependency create biased and pejorative representations of poor women. This work is an example of the immense political purchase that devolves from the postmodern understanding of language as a social accomplishment that constructs reality. Stories understood as radically vulnerable can be challenged and reauthored. Stories understood as objective reality demand passive acceptance:

> in a narrative, as you proceed along the narrative, the narrative takes on its own impetus as it were, so that one begins to see reality as non-narrated. One begins to say that it's not a narrative, it's the way things are.
>
> (Spivak, 1990: 19)

The authors in this volume demonstrate their refusals of dominant narratives as 'given' by pointing to other stories which may carry greater potential for social justice.

In case we are tempted to dismiss the claim that postmodernism is a crisis for social work as a grandiose overstatement, let us contrast the notion that social work knowledge consists of stories that are radically vulnerable with the hegemonic understanding of social work knowledge. The last century witnessed the uncritical adoption of standards of scientific methods as guarantees of truth. Schools of social work subsumed knowledge creation into a paradigm that accepts the possibility that there can be knowledge that is independent of the knower. This idea assumes an objective reality that proper methods can accurately describe, where such methods eliminate the 'bias' of the observer. This paradigm has dominated social work education, notwithstanding the emergence of qualitative research as the numerically challenged cousin of quantitative research. Consider the radical distance between the postmodern and modern answer to the question 'How does social work know what it knows?' The modernist answer is that we know through application of scientific techniques and value-free measurement (Irving, 1994). A postmodernist response, however, can be found in Donna Haraway's reworking of the notion of objectivity: We can know only from the limited view provided to us by our social location and context, and that view can only become less partial as a result of exchanges with others who are differently located (Haraway, 1988). Again, we need to point out the democratizing potential of multiple voices contributing to shaping the social construction of reality which is part of the post-modern project.

This brings us to the problem of the subject as an aspect of the crisis of knowledge in social work initiated by the understanding of the constituting function of language. The subject of modernism depends on an 'individual–social dualism' (Henriques et al., 1984) in which the individual is posited as having a pre-given self – a self that exists before socialisation. This pre-given self is an entity on which socialisation impresses itself. In other words, there is an essential self which exists outside the social and which is the basis for humanism. Such a formulation constructs a distinction between the individual and the social. In contrast, postmodernism sees the individual in terms of subjectivity. Here, selfhood is an effect of discourse, which is always/already social. Such a conception generates a subject who is social, where subjectivity is not stable or unitary, but 'precarious, contradictory and in process constantly being reconstituted in discourse each time we think or speak' (Weedon, 1987: 33).

Self as subjectivity has important implications for the political projects of feminism and social work. Feminism's hope is that if subjectivity is an effect of discourse, then there is no such thing as an immutable, essential femininity (Alcoff, 1988). Language and discourse, as socially constructed, can be politically contested and interrupted in service of emancipatory change. Social work builds on this insight chiefly through the demolition of the individual/social distinction. If the individual is always under social construction, then our attention to the individual must be based on an analysis of how the subject is constructed within multiple and intersecting discursive regimes.

The idea of a socially constructed subjectivity has far-reaching implications for the issue of difference. If there is no essential 'woman', and if each individual's particular location at the intersection of multiple discourses constitutes identity, then we must understand the subject as 'a site of differences ... that remain concretely embedded in social and power relations'. (de Lauretis, 1986: 14). This understanding represents an attack on the unifying and homogenising influences derived from the liberal humanist subject. The latter conception has its expression in social work theories and models which attempt to create unified perceptions of clients. Such unity is implicated in domination as it fails to acknowledge difference. As well, these strategies of unification fail to offer a nuanced description of the relations between subjectivity and power in the local and particular circumstances of clients' lives (Fook, 1995).

The possibility of a theory that refuses distinctions between the individual and the social has rich resonance for social work. Social work distinguishes its professional jurisdiction from other human services by its concern for 'persons in environments'. However, it has inherited Enlightenment theories based in liberal humanism that are predicated on the separation of the individual and the social. This theoretical impasse for social work has produced social work as an artefact of the individual–social distinction. Social work has teetered between emphases on the correction of internal landscapes of individuals or families, and insistence on correcting social environments in which individuals are located. Postmodern feminism offers a retheorisation of the individual as an effect of the social. This creates a space for social work to radically review its commitment to 'persons in environments', and has, in our view, the potential to unify social work as a democratic project. It also initiates important debates for social work concerning the nature of human agency and the extent to which the social 'determines' subjectivity.

The crisis of identity

The challenges to knowledge which devolve from postmodern feminism do not implicate only knowledge, leaving the knowers intact. Indeed, the very opposite is true: the crisis of knowledge takes us to a crisis of identity, which, although tremendously destabilising for the profession of social work, carries seeds for renewal of its ethical/political projects.

The crisis of identity has its roots in the postmodern turn regarding language. In the previous section, we discussed the notion of language as a social accomplishment rather than a medium which gives access to a reality 'out there'. The importance of this conception is that it locates languages within relations of power, for if language is social, then the power relations of the social construct language.

In our view, the heart of the postmodern project is its constant attention to the problem of power. Modernism tended to describe power in terms of force, or through discussions of legitimate versus illegitimate power. With postmodern theory, particularly through the work of Michel Foucault, power is relocated from specific and discrete social sites to everyday social relations. It is difficult to overestimate the significance of Foucault's work to social work and feminism.

Nancy Fraser describes Foucault's contribution as a 'a new form of politically engaged reflection on the emergence and nature of modern societies' (1989: 17). Fraser describes Foucault's genealogies in which he traces the development of forms of modern power. The features of Foucault's genealogies include his insistence that power is 'productive' rather than 'repressive' – it does more than inhibit – it produces forms, knowledges, categories which are the shapes of power. Foucault describes power as capillary, in that power is diffused throughout the social body, rather than concentrated in state formations. Power is exercised in 'micropractices' – or the everyday, ordinary patterns of daily life.

Foucault was interested to trace the development of modern power particularly through genealogies of the human sciences. In this work, he articulated the notion of 'power/knowledge relations' (Foucault, 1980), in which he understood that knowledge, operating through discourse, is inseparable from power. The aspect of power/knowledge relations that is most applicable to social work is Foucault's discussion of dividing practices (Foucault, 1984). Dividing practices are 'modes of manipulation that combine the mediation of a science (or pseudo-science) and the practice of exclusion' (Foucault, 1984: 8). Such modes of exclusion are obtained through objectification of subjects and through scientific classification.

In essence, Foucault understood the human sciences, of which social work is an outgrowth, as part of a web of power which formed new modes of government. Historical recourse to force and repressions no longer worked as modern society developed, and modes of power that relied on self-discipline, on unforced obedience were required. New modes of subjectification were achieved through classifications of deviance, criminality, or insanity. With such classifications, the regulation of populations through the establishment of 'normality' was achieved.

Foucault's harsh legacy for social work is the lost innocence of helping. Creating categories, administering correction, assessing under the approval of science, social work is inescapably organised by, even as it organises, modern power. However, its inheritance from modernism suggests the opposite – that the power to define is neutral, and its constitution of the Other is given by fact. Of modernism's binary thinking that organises social relations and conceals relations of domination, Jane Flax (1992) says the following. Her description is directly applicable to worker/client relations as relations of domination in social work:

> The superior member of the pair maintains his innocence. Unlike the inferior he is secure in his independence and natural superiority; he is within but not of the dyad. Like Aristotle's master or husband, his is the active matter, determining and generative within, but never affected by his coupling. There is no disorder within him and hence none within Being as such, but there may be disorderly objects requiring the exercise of his mastery. In the Enlightenment self-understanding, this view is an 'optimistic', humane and 'progressive' one; eventually all difference/disorder will be brought within the beneficent sovereignty of the One.
>
> (Flax, 1992: 454)

The relevance of Foucault's work for the human sciences becomes clear in his conception of 'governmentality'. Foucault talks about governmentality as 'a domain of strategic relations focusing on the behaviour of the other or others, and employing various procedures and techniques according to the case, the institutional frameworks, social groups and historical periods in which they develop' (Foucault, 1994: 88). What he means here is that the management of populations occurs through conceptions of self which are given in knowledge/power relations and disseminated by professionals who are authorised as knowing the 'truth'. The endpoint of governmentality is the 'docile body' (Foucault, 1979) who practise self-control as if she/he is individually motivated rather than governed.

The work of governmentality is done through exclusion. The human sciences have created categories, languages, and programmes which unify diverse people and place them on the margins as Other. People thus marginalised do the work of making the difference – of providing the contrast by which the centre, the authorised versions come into view. An understanding of governmentality requires analysis that 'attends to the "marginal" and shows its centrality, to the pathological as the condition for normality, to that considered inessential to show how, through it, the essential has been fabricated' (Rose, 1996: 80). What human sciences have created is a system of exclusions through which we can understand and induce the 'normal'.

Such a critique stands in stark contrast to social work's self-understanding. Social work educators are faced every year with waves of students who 'just want to help'. Their popular understanding of social work leaves no room for an analysis of power relations in social work. The profession itself has a long history of extolling its beneficence. Even radical social work has professed a space of innocence when it offers the choice of 'being an agent of social change or being an agent of social control'. This view suggests that there is a position to be found in social work that is somehow outside of power relations, rather than always as an effect of power.

Postmodern feminism suggests that to consider anything as outside of power is itself a 'ruse of authority' (Butler, 1992: 8). Social work has barely begun the work of understanding its construction within power. It still relies on notions of innocent helping by dedicated professionals to legitimate its presence. Leslie Margolin rather crudely interrupts social work's self-conception when he says 'social work stabilizes middle-class power by creating an observable, discussable, write-about-able poor' (1997: 6). Margolin goes on to describe social work's power to define reality, and in so doing, classify and extinguish difference: 'When social work describes its clients one way, all the other infinite ways those clients could be described are excluded. When social work establishes one reality, it necessarily blocks others; it is both positive and negative simultaneously' (ibid.: 7).

We might identify a more charitable description of the dilemma postmodernism poses for social work: There is no help that is outside governmentality. In working with marginalised people, social work contributes to cementing oppressive categories of marginality in service of supporting the centre. It is this challenge that creates a crisis of identity for social work. Postmodernism is, as Jane Flax puts it, 'the end of innocence' (Flax, 1992).

Feminist postmodernism, social work and radical democracy

What claims can we make regarding the contributions of postmodern feminism to social work? In our view, the force of postmodern feminism makes itself felt in social work in two profound ways: its analysis of power, and its insistence on difference.

At heart, postmodern feminism creates a demand in social work for deep self-reflexivity about the problem of power. North American social work, particularly its clinical versions, evolved from a history that virtually ignored the problem of power, favouring instead, models of individual pathology which hoped to explain deviance. Where critiques of this kind of social work existed, notably from structural social work, the problem of power was naively conceived through good/bad binaries. The indelible mark of postmodern feminism confronts social work with its responsibility to acknowledge power in the construction of social problems, and in its complicity with the process of construction. It demands acknowledgement of social work's own construction in power as well as that of its clients.

The challenge for social work is to determine how such reflection can produce a progressive political direction as opposed to an inevitable entrapment in complicity. Adrienne Chambon points to the potential offered by postmodernism for 'stepping outside of the very institutions' which we form in order to examine the constituting effects of changing language and discourse on social work's direction (1994: 71). Such a practice is, in Foucault's terms a 'practice of freedom' (Foucault, 1997: 284) in that it enables conscious resistance to the operation of power. In Chambon's terms 'a reflexive orientation would imply the re-examination of the terminology and narratives that constitute our practice, as a prevention measure against creeping heteronomy' (Chambon, 1994: 71).

Such a reflexive orientation will require social work to raise new questions about the meaning of social work as an effect of power. A central question involves the problem that helping a marginalised group also serves to construct it. How do we find ways to help marginalised people which ensuring that we resist the creating of homogenising categories of exclusion which support reigning conceptions of the centre? How can we confront the question Karen Healy poses concerning the difference between power and domination (Healy, 1998)?

Taking the problem of power seriously encourages a much more complex reflection on the operation of power through us and through our clients. Understanding that there is no knowledge independent of the knower abolishes an easy recourse to models and schemas for decoding human behaviour. Instead, a postmodern social work insists that social workers are socially located in particular historical and social spaces, and that their knowledge is a partial perspective that is tied to their social location. Workers cannot obliterate their presence in knowledge through universal prescriptions. Instead, Jane Gorman suggests that workers are obliged to engage in self-reflection in order to understand how their own 'biases, needs, prejudices, values, expectations and life experiences' form the conditions and the limitations of hearing clients' narratives (1993: 262).

Postmodern feminism also contributes a perspective which allows social work to develop analyses which do not depend on the bifurcation of the individual and social and which do not flow from grand narratives of human behaviour. This allows for specific, concrete, and local understandings with room for the kind of complexity that characterises lived experience. Featherstone and Fawcett (1995) point to this advantage, saying that the rejection of grand narratives means:

> the development of analyses which explored specific situations and located them and those who studied them, in relation to class, gender, culture, ethnicity, rather than analyses which started from abstract or universal notions of childhood or abuse ... This could assist in the process of moving away from di-

chotomous thinking, towards perspectives which can encompass the possibility that problems exist on a number of levels.
(Featherstone and Fawcett, 1995: 36)

The lesson from postmodernism concerning the tendency of grand narratives to exclude by denying difference takes us to the necessity for social work to come to terms with difference. It is clear that the grand narratives of social work install 'the client' as a projection of middle-class white imagination while simultaneously eliminating difference through recourse to values concerning universal human subjects. Postmodern feminism leaves us with a version of human subjects as diverse, socially constructed from different cultural locations, and multiply positioned with respect to social identities.

Such an analysis has great value for contemporary social work. Many of us find ourselves doing social work in a radically changed global context. We who work in the West confront the history of colonisation when new immigrant populations require culturally appropriate social work services or when social workers of non-dominant ethnicity confront their exclusion in the professional system. Here, the shattering of the universal subject opens the possibility that we can create a decentred solidarity based on a kind of multicultural pluralism. This ideal is a very long way from the recent history of human sciences, which created individual deficits and pathologies from differences due to race, class, gender and sexual orientation.

We are arguing, then, that a social work allied with postmodern feminism enables reflexivity about power which inheres in social work, and that questions about power have opened up new space for understanding and celebrating difference. Is this enough to renew social work as a political project? While we have argued above that elements of postmodernist feminism have a profoundly democratising influence on social work, recent feminist work calls for augmenting a postmodem sensibility with a politics of solidarity. Under the general rubric of radical democracy (Trend, 1996), the necessity for a post-Marxist political project requires uniting postmodem feminism with political goals. Here, Selya Benhabib (1996) argues for a 'social feminism' which redresses the fragmenting tendencies of identity politics. In a similar vein, Nancy Fraser says that 'we must find a way to combine the struggle for an anti-essentialist multiculturalism with the struggle for social equality'

(1996: 206). Fraser insists that both anti-essentialism and multiculturalism must understand that 'cultural differences can only be freely elaborated and democratically mediated on the basis of social equality' (ibid., 207). Surely social work has deep resonance with the call to create political solidarity alongside the pluralism and anti-essentialism that have destabilised relations of domination. As we struggle in local and particular social work contexts, what will help us to know that we are also struggling for social justice? How will we know the difference between justice and injustice? Is there a next step for social work that will allow us to 'move beyond identity politics, in the Hegelian sense of moving beyond (*Aufheben*), that is, by learning its lessons, rejecting its excesses, and moving to a new synthesis of collective solidarities with plurally constituted identities' (Benhabib, 1996: 38)?

Bibliography

Alcoff, L. (1988) 'Cultural feminism versus post-structuralism: the identity crisis in feminist theory', *Signs* 13(3): 405–36.

Benhabib, S. (1996) 'From identity politics to social feminism: a plea for the nineties', in D. Trend (ed.) *Radical Democracy: Identity. Citizenship and the State*, New York: Routledge.

Butler, J. (1992) 'Contingent foundations: feminism and the question of postmodernism', in J. Butler and J. Scott (eds) *Feminists Theorise the Political*, New York: Routledge.

Chambon, A. (1994) 'Postmodernity and social work discourses: notes on the changing language of a profession', in A. Chambon and A. Irving (eds) *Essays on Postmodernism and Social Work*, Toronto: Canadian Scholar's Press.

de Lauretis, T. (1986) 'Feminist studies/critical studies: issues, terms, and contexts', in T. de Lauretis (ed.) *Feminist Studies/Critical Studies*, Bloomington, Indiana University Press.

Dews, P. (1989) 'The return of the subject in late Foucault', *Radical Philosophy* 51 (Spring): 37–41.

Featherstone, B. and Fawcett, B. (1995) 'Oh no! Not more isms: feminism, postmodernism, poststructuralism, and social work education', *Social Work Education* Autumn, 15(1): 3–20.

Flax, J. (1990a) *Thinking Fragments: Psychoanalysis, Feminism, and Postmodernism in the Contemporary West*, Berkeley, CA: University of California Press.

—— (1990b) 'Postmodernism and gender relations in feminist theory', in N. Nicholson (ed.) *Feminism/Postmodernism*, New York: Routledge.

—— (1992) 'The end of innocence', in J. Butler and J. Scott (eds) *Feminists Theorise the Political*, New York: Routledge.

Fook, J. (1995) 'Beyond structuralism', paper presented at Monash University, Narratives of Social Change, November, Australia.

Foucault, M. (1979) *Discipline and Punish: The Birth of the Prison*, New York: Vintage.

—— (1980) *Power/Knowledge: Selected Interviews and Other Writings 1972 – 1977*, ed. C. Gordon, New York: Pantheon Books.

—— (1984) *The Foucault Reader*, ed. P. Rabinow, New York: Pantheon.

—— (1994) 'Subjectivity and truth', in P. Rabinow (ed.) *The Essential Works of Michel Foucault 1954–1984*, New York: The New Press.

—— (1997) *Ethics: Subjectivity and Truth*, ed. P. Rabinow, New York: The New Press.

Fraser, N. (1989) *Unruly Practices: Power, Discourse and Gender in Contemporary Social Theory*, Minneapolis: University of Minnesota Press.

—— (1996) 'Equality, difference, and radical democracy: the United States feminist debates revisited', in D. Trend (ed.) *Radical Democracy: Identity, Citizenship and the State*, New York: Routledge.

Fraser, N. and Gordon, L. (1994) 'Dependency demystified: inscriptions of power in a keyword of the welfare state', *Social Politics* Spring, 4–31.

Fraser, N. and Nicholson, L. (1990) 'Social criticism without philosophy: an encounter between feminism and postmodernism', in L. Nicholson (ed.) *Feminism/ Postmodernism*, New York: Routledge.

Gorman, J. (1993) 'Postmodernism and the conduct of inquiry in social work', *Affilia* 8(3): 247–64.

Haraway, D. (1988) 'Situated knowledges: the science question in feminism and the privilege of partial perspective', *Feminist Studies* 14(3): 575–99.

Healy, K. (1998) 'Activist social work', paper presented at Deakin University, Critical Social Work Research and Practice Conference, Geelong, Australia, November.

Henriques, J., Hollway, W., Urwin, C., Venn, C. and Walkerdine, V. (1984) *Changing the Subject: Psychology, Social Regulation and Subjectivity*, London: Methuen.

Irving, A. (1994) 'From image to simulacra: the modern/postmodern divide and social work', in A. Chambon and A. Irving (eds) *Essays on Postmodernism and Social Work*, Toronto: Canadian Scholars Press, pp. 19–32.

Leonard, P. (1994) 'Knowledge/power and postmodernism', *Canadian Social Work Review* 11(1): 11–26.

—— (1997) *Postmodern Welfare: Reconstructing an Emancipatory Project*, London: Sage.

Margolin, L. (1997) *Under the Cover of Kindness: The Invention of Social Work*, Charlottesville: University Press of Virginia.

Rose, N. (1996) *Inventing Ourselves: Psychology, Power, and Personhood*, Cambridge: Cambridge University Press.

Sands, R. and Nuccio, K. (1992) 'Postmodern feminist theory and social work', *Social Work* 37(6): 489–94.

Spivak, G. (1990) *The Postcolonial Critic: Interviews, Strategies, Dialogues*, New York: Routledge, Chapman and Hall.

Trend, D. (1996) 'Introduction', in D. Trend (ed.) *Radical Democracy: Identity, Citizenship and the State*, New York: Routledge.

Wapner, Paul (1989) 'What's left: Marx, Foucault and the contemporary problems of change', *Praxis International* 9(1/2): 88–111.

Weedon, C. (1987) *Feminist Practice and Poststructuralist Practice*, Oxford: Basil Blackwell.

Chapter 3

Reading the texts

Postmodern feminism and the 'doing' of research

Liz Trinder

Introduction

This chapter argues for the relevance of postmodern feminist perspectives for social work research. The main argument is that much social work research largely excludes consideration of gender issues (as well as many other forms of social relations), while much research which does engage with gender does so within a theoretical and epistemological framework which precludes consideration of the complexity of gender relations or their interconnection with other forms of social relations.

This chapter focuses on outlining broad trends within social work research. It begins by considering the largely gender-free approaches to research of empirical/evidence-based practice and pragmatism, then considers the mainly standpoint feminist approaches which characterise much of the social work research which does concern itself with gender issues. I will argue that the theoretical and epistemological insights of postmodern feminism have much to offer as a practice relevant and justice-orientated approach to social work research. The final section of the chapter draws on current developments within poststructuralist and postmodern approaches to research practice to outline some of the components of a possible postmodern feminism approach to social work research practice. The intention is not to suggest that a postmodern feminism informed research practice should replace other approaches. Even if that were a realistic prospect it would, I think, be undesirable. Other research approaches still have much to offer, but the development of a body of postmodern feminist informed theory and research practice is important in its own right as well as potentially generating a productive dialogue with other non-postmodern feminist approaches.

Three social work research trends

Research and evaluation have had a long but contested history in social work. Social workers were amongst the earliest to evaluate interventions. Nevertheless, the nature and role of research in social work have continued to generate intense and often acrimonious exchanges. Debates in both the United States and United Kingdom have frequently been polarised between experimental/empirical and non-experimental camps. Neither has concerned itself centrally or even marginally with gender issues or gender relations. Largely on the fringes, a body of radical/standpoint feminist-inspired research has built up. Although there have been attempts to reconcile differences, none the less the history of social work research is best characterised as heterogeneous with competing approaches to research running in parallel, each with particular periods of prominence.

In the following sections I examine in turn three major trends in social work research. In outline the three trends are:

1   *Empirical and evidence-based practice.* This is becoming increasingly prominent, particularly in probation work, in the United Kingdom. It is centred on positivist/post-positivist experimental methods and very limited attention is paid to gender.
2   *Pragmatism.* This is very prominent in the United Kingdom and involves working within a realist epistemological framework. It is primarily survey-based with some attention to gender.
3   *Critical/Standpoint.* This is relatively marginal in influence, drawing on critical theory especially radical feminism within a standpoint epistemological framework. It is primarily though not exclusively qualitative, with a central focus on gender.

Empirical and evidence-based practice

There is a long-standing tradition of experimental research in social work. The experimental tradition began in the USA in the 1930s with a major study on preventing delinquency (Powers and Witmer, 1951). The formation of the Social Work Research Group in the USA in the 1950 gave a further thrust to an experimental 'scientific' approach to social work based on the application of findings from randomised controlled trials (Tyson, 1995). Although the methodological approach was far from universally accepted, the substantive findings were highly influential as a succession of studies reported that social work methods were ineffective (e.g. Mullen and Dumpson, 1972; Segal, 1972; Fischer, 1973; Martinson, 1974; Lipton et al., 1975; Fischer, 1976; Folkard et al., 1976; Wood, 1978). For both social work and probation the 'nothing works' conclusion drawn from these experimental studies dealt a devastating blow to the self-esteem and rehabilitative ideals of a profession committed to helping people, and particularly to the dominant approach of psychoanalytic casework.

Over the last two decades the experimental approach positivist paradigm has been reframed and relaunched in social work, beginning in the United States as part of an identifiable empirical practice movement, and subsequently finding supporters in the United Kingdom (see Sheldon, 1986; Macdonald and Sheldon, 1992; Macdonald and Roberts, 1995; Macdonald, 1996). The background or rationale to this shift is a rejection of the critiques of the 1970s that 'nothing works', and a shift to attempts to prove that the right things (generally more structured methods of intervention such as cognitive-behavioural therapy) do work, at least if rigorously measured (e.g. Reid and Hanrahan, 1980, 1982; Rubin, 1985: Thomlinson, 1984; Videka-Sherman, 1988; Macdonald and Sheldon, 1992).

The empirical/evidence-based practice movement draws upon a positivist or post-positivist epistemological framework, that is there is an objective reality which exists which can, through rigorous and objective research, be captured. The methods associated with this approach are experimental ones (the randomised controlled trial (RCT) and single case designs). The central concern of this approach is testing the effectiveness of social work interventions. The only way to test and re-test whether or not an intervention works, is to conduct an RCT with an experimental design and randomly assigned control groups. Thus practice can and should be based on 'proven facts' generated through RCTs or single system/case evaluations, rather than 'less rigorous' research designs, intuition, practice wisdom or theory. Quasi-experimental designs (with a non-randomised control group), pre-experimental designs, client-opinion studies and surveys are simply not rigorous enough to evaluate effectiveness (see Sheldon, 1986; Macdonald and Sheldon,

1992; Macdonald and Roberts, 1995; Macdonald, 1996). In the United States, and to a much lesser degree in the United Kingdom, considerable emphasis has also been placed on single system single case experiments conducted by practitioner researchers to evaluate effectiveness (for American sources see Hersen and Barlow, 1976; Bloom and Block, 1977; Blythe and Briar, 1985, Thyer and Thyer, 1992; Bloom, 1993, and for a British advocate see Sheldon, 1983). Here the single case/system acts as its own control with comparisons drawn between baseline measures and post-intervention outcome measures (AB), or, more rigorously, with additional measurements post-withdrawal and repeat of an intervention (ABAB).

Over the last few years the indigenous social work empirical practice movement in the United Kingdom has gained further momentum by explicitly linking with the evidence-based practice movement originating within medicine (see for example Sackett *et al.*, 1996, 1997). Both share a concern with basing practice upon hard empirical data generated through RCTs. The two most prominent advocates of empirical practice in the UK, Geraldine Macdonald and Brian Sheldon, have explicitly adopted the 'evidence-based' tag. Macdonald, has written extensively, if at times despairingly, of the need for RCTs and evidence-based social work (1997a, b). Brian Sheldon now heads up a new Centre for Evidence-Based Social Services with funding from the Department of Health and social services departments. In probation work a recent Home Office practice guide significantly entitled *Evidence-Based Practice: A Guide to Effective Practice* (Home Office, 1998) draws heavily on RCT and meta-analysis findings on interventions to reduce offending. A national implementation strategy for this 'Effective Practice Initiative' is currently underway, including revision of National Standards binding on all probation officers.

Positivism and the use of RCTs in social work research have been subject to sustained criticism, largely on the grounds that the complexity of human relations and interventions cannot be captured by the rigour or rigidity of experimental methods and that the epistemological and methodological framework are far from neutral but contain an unacknowledged world view seeing human subjects as ordered, rational and autonomous beings (see Smith, 1987; Witkin, 1996; Trinder, 1996, 1999). Rather than rehearse these arguments here, what is more germane to this particular discussion is to recognise the virtual exclusion of gender from this approach. Where gender, or more accurately 'sex' does appear, it is solely within the context of a rigidly defined male/female binary considered as an independent variable influencing the dependent variable. Thus the technology of the RCT of empirical or evidence-based practice gives us limited purchase on gender or gender relations.

Pragmatism

In the UK most research, and most research on social work effectiveness, fits within a broad pragmatist approach. Much of the non-experimental research on effectiveness and many of the researchers who have participated in Department of Health (hereafter DoH) funded childcare and social care research would fall into this category (see Cheetham *et al.*, 1992; Fuller and Petch, 1995; Dartington Social Research Unit, 1995). Though the pragmatists are not formally united by a manifesto in the same way as the empirical practice movement there is a significant degree of *de facto* commonality, including broadly shared views on social work practice, research design, methods and epistemology. Grand science and grand experimental designs are cut down to size within a realist epistemological framework. For Fuller this means 'the suspension of not-to-be resolved philosophical conundra in the interests of getting on with the job' (1996: 59), leading to a trade-off between what is desirable and what is feasible, and abandoning the search for irrefutable scientific proof (ibid.). Epistemological discussions and theory are not part of pragmatism, and the pragmatists appear to continue to exist in splendid isolation from developments and debates in research methodology outside of social work. For pragmatists research design is therefore based on technical rather than epistemological, ontological or theoretical grounds. There is a strong preference for non-experimental quantitative methods of data collection using non-randomised samples, or quasi-experimental, comparing areas or pre-post-test. A classic pragmatist design would include surveys, file searches, and some psychological tests. Qualitative methods for data collection are frequently incorporated in a secondary or supplementary role. Where qualitative methods are used, they tend to be fairly structured, for example, semi-structured interviewing rather than depth interviews or observation.

The main task of pragmatic research for Fuller (1996: 59) 'is to study social work as it is'. Pragmatic research designs have greatly contributed to our understanding of social work interventions, but have been restricted to asking certain types of questions. The 'what social work is' tends to be what is visible or evident. Research questions are descriptive and evaluative – how is the system working, and what are the outcomes? In terms of gender there is some consideration of gender issues but it is very limited.

Critical/standpoint research

Critical/standpoint research differs from empirical practice and pragmatist research in two key and related ways, first, it has an explicit gender focus informed by radical feminism, and second, a belief that research is about politics and change rather than attempts at dispassionate neutral recording. For critical/standpoint researchers the research act, like social work practice, is about power and empowerment. Research is not posited as a neutral fact-finding activity. Instead, research, researchers and research participants are located within a world where power is unequally distributed between genders. Lives and life-stories are significantly structured by these unequal power relations, with significant implications for uncovering 'truths'. Research can therefore be used to ignore, reinforce or, preferably for critical/standpoint researchers, to identify and challenge inequalities. To achieve the latter there is a strong emphasis on using research findings to identify power relations, specifically the oppression of women. Feminist research in social work and surrounding disciplines has therefore focused on specific subject areas, especially the issue of men's violence against women and children.

In terms of methods, much critical/standpoint research is qualitative. There is some emphasis in the feminist methodological literature on collaborative and non-hierarchical approaches to research with the researcher attempting to involve participants (usually service users/front-line professionals) in the research process (e.g. Everitt et al., 1992; Hart and Bond, 1995; Everitt and Hardiker, 1996). Although there is a strong emphasis on qualitative research within this tradition there has also been some important quantitative work, including a number of studies on the incidence of men's violence (see, for example, Kelly et al., 1991).

What unites the range of researchers in this approach then is not method but a shared theoretical understanding committed to uncovering and challenging women's oppression. Crucially this is typically framed in terms of giving women 'a voice', something which society in general and researchers in particular are accused of ignoring or suppressing. Allied to this is an implicit or explicit commitment to the particular epistemological framework of feminist standpoint theory. Feminist standpoint theorists believe that the standpoint of women and of feminism is less partial and distorted than the picture of nature and social relations that emerges from conventional 'malestream' research (Harding, 1991). In terms of research practices, radical feminists have largely adopted standpoint approaches. It is not just that women have a different understanding of the world, but that it is a better understanding. The grounds for this claim lie in the distinctiveness of women's emotional and material lives (see Swigonski, 1993 on standpoint and social work research).

In terms of the violence literature, two related claims are made: that women's voices or experiences must be heard, and that these experiences represent a privileged insight into reality. An example of a particular research project might be helpful. Hester and Radford's (1996) study of non-residential fathers having contact with their children concluded that contact puts both mother and child at risk of violence.[1] The researchers found that professionals had a 'poor awareness' of domestic violence, and (unfairly) perceived mothers as hostile to contact when in fact mothers were acting upon concerns for their own and their children's safety. The study was based on interviews with mothers, professionals and two children. The presumption was, consistent with standpoint theory, that women's experience is authentic, true and sufficient. Children's experiences and wishes (with two exceptions) were represented by their mothers. No men were interviewed. Men's experiences were excluded on the grounds that domestic violence is mainly committed by men on women (Hester and Radford, 1996: 53).

The Hester and Radford study, indeed critical/standpoint research as a whole, has performed a vital function in highlighting issues which have been neglected by both practitioners and researchers. These include the prevalence and impact of sexual abuse, domestic violence and sexual harassment. This work has made an impact. In domestic violence, in particular, even what would be seen as non-feminist organisations are responding to the issue and using the framework provided by standpoint researchers (see, for example, National Children's Homes Action for Children, 1994; Social Services Inspectorate, 1995).

Yet there are significant problems with this approach. Flax (1990, 1993), amongst others, has criticised standpoint approaches, arguing that they conflate three claims. One claim is that certain kinds of knowledge are generated by gender-based power relations. The second, is that they then go on to argue that better knowledge is produced by feminists, and third, that this knowledge is straightforwardly emancipatory and does not generate its own power relations. The first of these is justifiable, the second and third are not.

The contact and domestic violence research illustrates some of the claims Flax identifies, as well as the problems which ensue. Although the discussion which follows is based on a single piece of research, it can be taken as illustrating much of the critical/standpoint research.

The dilemma of standpoint theory, however, is that the three claims are mutually contradictory. If, as Harding herself acknowledges, women's experiences are shaped by (gendered) social relations (claim one), then women's experiences in themselves, or the things women say, cannot provide reliable grounds for knowledge claims about nature and social relations:

> After all, experience itself is shaped by social relations: for example, women have had to learn to define as rape those sexual assaults that occur within marriage. Women had experienced these assaults not as something which could be called rape but only as part of the range of heterosexual sex that wives should expect.
>
> (Harding 1991: 123)

For a position to count as a standpoint, rather than a claim, we must insist, Harding argues, on an objective location from which feminist research can begin which she terms 'women's lives'. It is not the experience or the speech that provides the grounds for feminist claims, but the subsequently articulated observations of, and theory about, the rest of nature and social relations; these observations start out from and look from the perspective of women's lives (1991: 124). Kelly, a prominent researcher on violence follows suit, arguing that taking an explicitly feminist standpoint implies looking at the world from the standpoint of women, but that 'given that most knowledge has been created from men's point of view and that women as well as men have been encouraged to accept this knowledge as having a universal applicability, women can and often do, see the world through men's eyes' (Kelly, 1992: 108). As Smart (1992) notes not just any experience is deemed to be equally valid or valuable. Rather, it is feminist experience which is achieved through a struggle against oppression which is more complete and less distorted.

Hester and Radford's study on contact demonstrates some of the problems which ensue with such an approach. The contact study gives an interesting if confusing account of the role of experience, or whether it is women's or feminist definitions which are important. The researchers do not, at least explicitly, offer their own definition of domestic violence. What happens instead is that a composite definition of domestic violence is given which is represented as being based on the women's experiences and one which exactly mirrors radical feminist understandings of domestic violence. This definition is therefore rendered powerful and one which is morally empowered to judge other definitions. Professional definitions or understandings of domestic violence are compared with what has become the 'true' understanding of domestic violence, rendering some definitions 'correct': 'refuge workers, and to a lesser extent solicitors, had perceptions of domestic violence that most closely reflected the experiences outlined by the women' (Hester and Radford, 1996: 11). While others were therefore 'incorrect' definitions of domestic violence:

> Nearly all the solicitors saw domestic violence as involving a range of abuse of differing degrees of severity, women's concerns escalating with the degree of severity. In this respect there tended to be an *overemphasis* on physical violence compared to women's accounts.
>
> (1996: 12, my emphasis)

A further problem with the study is the unitariness or total coherence of the women's accounts. Hollway (1989) argues that all research accounts are productions in a particular time and space. She argues that there is no context, however private and searching, which would provide the account which tells the whole truth as the number of possible accounts is infinite. Accounts must be seen as provisional and incomplete, recognising the infinite number of things that were not said. In the Hester and Radford study the unitariness of the account, the lack of any contrary evidence to men's utter complicity and women's utter innocence makes one wonder about the extent to which the voices of the women interviewees are presented in all their complexity or whether they have been (even unconsciously) filtered by a feminist understanding of domestic violence.

Allied to this is the unitariness of the subject positions represented in the account. Smart (1992) argues that because standpoint feminism arises from a grass roots concern to protect women and to reveal the victimisation of women, it has not been sympathetic to the study of men and masculinity. The Hester and Radford study on contact presents a telling example of this. Both gender and generational categories are understood as comprising a set of opposite and inherently different beings with unitary constant and consistent selves. The gender identities in this script are familiarly unitary, discrete and oppositional. Men are produced as a monolithic brutalising other, appearing only as woman/child abusers, never as nurturers or carers. Women are the victims of abusive men, always done to rather than doing, but nevertheless fierce protectors of their children. Children are presented as an undifferentiated category of vulnerable and largely passive victims, at risk not only of abuse but also manipulation by their fathers.

This brings us to the central tension in critical/standpoint research, that is how to retain the centrality of the subject (the informant) and their voices while recognising the constructed nature of social relations and differential power relations. In much standpoint research this dilemma is resolved by smoothing out complexity, working with fixed oppositional subject categories and eliding women's voices and feminist consciousness. But a series of questions remain:

- What is the status of the account?
- Are the voices of women (or other oppressed groups) true or more true than others?
- How should we judge truth claims?

Elsewhere, there is considerable interest and continuing debate about these major epistemological questions, drawing on constructivism and poststructuralism and postmodernism which we will consider below. Within the feminist social work research body is some recognition that these issues are important and that standpoint theory may be insufficient, but as yet the answers are unconvincing.

Everitt and Hardiker (1996), for example, argue that researchers should make a fundamental shift away from seeking the truth, and towards researching how truths are produced or how things come to be seen as true (ibid.: 105). Drawing on poststructuralist and postmodern theory they argue that knowledge is not neutral, disinterested and socially beneficial, but represents a claim to power. Researchers, so Everitt and Hardiker (ibid: 106) argue, should examine how discourses ('texts, languages, behaviours, a multitude of policies and practices') construct subjects and what we know and how we come to be known. Everitt and Hardiker go on to examine the work of Nancy Fraser (1989) on how need is discursively constituted in a multitude of ways, and how different versions of 'needs-talk' become authoritative while others are marginalised. So

'Evaluation becomes a dialogical process providing opportunities for all, practitioners and users alike, to reflect upon and understand the meaning of their experiences. This is with a view to deepening those understandings to take account of ways in which they have been shaped through discourses.
(Everitt and Hardiker, 1996: 151)

Unfortunately Everitt and Hardiker (1996) still have too strong a foothold in critical theory to follow through with their own analysis. In practice, the focus of their energies is on challenging managerial non-participatory styles of evaluation by getting suppressed (users') voices heard through democratic research processes (e.g. ibid.: 152, 177, 179). Thus the primary task is to make 'emancipatory truth claims' (ibid.: 1), and not asking the question of why people are saying what they say. The commitment to participation and a particular mode of challenging oppression remains paramount, and trumps the focus on uncovering how truths come to be established. Implicitly we are back to standpoint theory where the voices of the oppressed have a privileged status.

There is therefore a fundamental contradiction between moving the subject centre stage and attempting to analyse how subjects are discursively created, and how 'truths' come to be established as 'truths'. The contradiction arises for Everitt and Hardiker because they adopt a radical postmodern epistemological framework alongside concepts of power, subjectivity, gender and oppression derived from critical theory. Thus, for them, user involvement means people being 'confident to speak on their own terms, being respected as subjects in their own right' (Everitt and Hardiker 1996: 178). Despite their calls for deconstruction of accounts, they remain reluctant to examine why 'the oppressed' say what they say, or how gendered discourses are sustained or resisted.

Poststructuralist/postmodern feminism and research practice

One route out of the tension between deconstruction and empowerment is offered by postmodern feminism. Previous chapters have outlined the major concerns of postmodern feminism, including an interest in the historically and socially situated self, subjectivity and an emphasis on gender relations as forms of domination, but ones with no fixed pattern. For postmodern feminism the focus shifts therefore away from feminist theorising with clear-cut notions of oppressors and victims to interrogating how masculinities and femininities are constructed and operate in relation to each other. Men, women, boys and girls are located within systems where expectations around roles and responsibilities are sites of struggle and definition.

What does this mean for research practice? What should be researched? How should research be judged? There has been a considerable amount of development and debate on these questions in poststructuralist and postmodernist influenced work on research over the last decade (see, for example, Denzin and Lincoln, 1994), much of which is relevant to postmodern feminist research practice. In the following section I will introduce some of this work, considering in turn what is to be researched, how it can be researched and how research can be evaluated. In the final section I consider some of the possible criticisms of postmodern feminist research practice.

What is to be researched?

The 'rhetorical or linguistic turn' in social sciences over the last decade has introduced a shift from seeing language as referring to a concrete reality to seeing language as constructive of reality (Filmer *et al.*, 1998:24). In terms of research practice the focus then shifts away from postpositivist frameworks predicated on an assumption of an external reality or interpretivism seeking the research participant's own reality, characteristic of symbolic interactionist approaches to qualitative research. Instead, poststructuralist and postmodernist research has adopted a relativist ontology based on a presumption of local specific constructed realities, with constructions not more or less 'true', in any absolute sense, but simply more or less informed and/or sophisticated. This raises two key issues, first, whether lived experience can be directly captured untainted by social relations (the representational crisis) and, second, if all truth claims are knowledge claims, again within language, how then can research be interpreted and evaluated (see Denzin, 1994; Denzin and Lincoln, 1994a, b; Guba and Lincoln, 1994).

The implication of this is not nihilistic. Researchers should not simply give up, but language, or discourse, itself becomes the object of study. As Hollway (1989: 40) argues, research can and should focus on the discourses research participants are using to position themselves at the time. For postmodern feminist researchers a particular interest then will be an analysis of the gendered discourses research participants use in particular locations at particular times, as well as the intersection with other discourses. This shifts us away from a reified and fixed notions of 'woman' or 'man'. It also moves us away from attempting to articulate or capture women's voices to examining what voices women (and men) are using within the context of unequal gender and other social relations.

How might postmodern feminist research be undertaken?

Research practice which conceptualises the world in terms of a range of discursive resources available to individuals and groups has two important consequences. First, it problematises the notion that researchers can, by building empathy and trust, reliably access true and singular perspectives and experiences through, for example, the interview. Instead within poststructuralist and postmodern research practice the interview is seen not as a straightforward window on the world, the interviewees' 'true' feelings, but as a local accomplishment, a topic in its own right, where the researcher uses the interview to examine both which discursive resources or linguistic repertoires the interviewee draws upon, what moral reputation or self-identity is displayed and how accounts are constructed within that particular context (Potter and Mulkay, 1985; Riessman, 1993; Silverman, 1993: Chapter 5; Seale, 1998).

The second consequence is that the interpretive role of the researcher at all stages of the research process is given greater definition. Just as the interpretive role of research participants is highlighted in poststructuralist and postmodernist research, so too is that of the researcher in gathering data, in the process of transcription of data, in analysis, and in the representational form within which findings are presented (Riessman, 1993; Van Maanen, 1988).

Two approaches which take up some of these themes – analytic narrative analysis and discourse analysis – will now be briefly outlined. They are not the only ways of doing poststructuralist or postmodernist research but they do illustrate some of the themes which characterise this form of research practice. Neither could be explicitly described as postmodern feminist research practice but both can, informed by postmodern feminist theory provide some of the foundations for postmodern feminist research.

Analytic narrative analysis

Catherine Riessman, an American social work academic, argues that narratives are a universal form of particular relevance to researchers (see Riessman, 1990, 1993, 1994). Narratives or stories are a primary way in which social actors make sense of past experiences, giving a view of past events as well as the meaning subsequently attributed to those events. The presumption is that meaning is not fixed or universal but fluid and contextual. Accounts are told in and shaped by a particular context, produced interactionally with the interview as one example. Riessman argues that narratives are not random but highly structured drawing on a range of (often gendered) cultural or public meanings, of, for example, divorce or marital violence. Thus accounts are always evolving and never concluded as private and public meanings shift. A crucial aspect of narrative analysis, as in other forms of poststructuralist and postmodernist research, is the idea that the form of the narrative is related to the content. The key tasks of the narrative analyst are therefore to analyse how a narrative is structured, the linguistic and cultural resources it draws on, and how it persuades a listener of authenticity. According to Riessman, research participants:

> create who they are, and definitions of their divorce situations, in interaction and through language … There is a reciprocity between form and function, that is, between the way an account is told (how it is narrated), the understandings the narrator wants to convey, and the listening process.
>
> (1990: 74)

To illustrate, Riessman (1990) identified different types of narratives in her own research on divorce, distinguished by structure, codes of speech including verb tense, temporality, sequencing and rhetorical devices including metaphor, contrast and repetition. In an 'episodic story' for example the narrative was held together thematically rather than temporally with three episodes of marital violence/rape used to make a general point about male/female power imbalances. In contrast, a 'habitual story' about an unsatisfying frustrating marriage described the general course of events over time rather than recalling specific incidents. The narrative persuades the listener by 'recreating' the quality of the marriage, where the structure and rhetorical devices within the narrative convey a sense of time dragging.

Discourse analysis

Discourse analysis shares many of the same concerns as narrative analysis though the focus is less on the individual as in narrative analysis and more on discursive resources or interpretive repertoires expressed in a variety of texts – in documents, film, magazine as well as interviews. Again language is viewed not as a neutral medium for conveying information but as a mean by which the social world is constituted, where meaning is created and reproduced and social identities formed (Tonkiss, 1998; Potter and Wetherell, 1995; Gill, 1996; Potter, 1996).

Gill (1996: 141–2) summarises the themes of discourse analysis as follows:

- An interest in discourse as interesting in its own right, rather than what lies behind it or what people 'really' think.

- Language is constructive. People 'choose' from a range of pre-existing linguistic resources or discourses.
- Discourse has an action or function orientation. People choose discourse in order to DO things, such as offer blame, make excuses or present themselves in the best possible light. Thus all discourse is occasioned within a particular interpretive context (including gender) and so the discourses use will change in different contexts (with a family member compared to a social worker, for example).
- Talk and texts are rhetorically organised to make themselves persuasive in the face of other competing ac counts.

Discourse analysis research typically begins with a broad open research question. In an interview study each interview will be carefully and fully transcribed, including pauses and emphasis. The text will then be read and reread before being sorted into relevant sections. Analysis is based on a search for patterns within the data crucially both of consistency and inconsistency rather than attempting to summarise the gist of what seemed to be intended, and on the rhetorical organisation of the text (including rhetorical devices and appeal to particular discourses).

Evaluating research

The evaluation of particular pieces of research is contested. Different research traditions – positivist/post-positivist, interpretivist, critical theory and post-structuralist and postmodern – all have different criteria for judging the quality of research. In contrast to positivist or post-positivist research with very clear criteria for assessing research, or interpretivist and critical theory which have some criteria, for post-structuralist and postmodern research there are no agreed criteria, indeed, given the emphasis on discourse and a relativist epistemology, it is unlikely that there could or should be.

That is not to say that all research is equally good or equally bad. From a discourse analysis perspective Potter (1996: 138–9) emphasises the importance of deviant-case analysis (searching for data which contradicts expectations or hypotheses), a close attention to participants' understandings, the coherence of an account, and the presentation of data to enable readers to make their own evaluation. Riessman (1993) considers a number of suggestions including reflexivity (the researchers question their own assumptions and processes of inquiry and consider their effect on the research), the persuasiveness of the account and the extent to which a piece of research is used by other researchers. None of these suggestions, she adds, are ultimately conclusive or guarantees of 'truth'.

There are, however, no agreed standards for evaluating poststructuralist or postmodernist research. The criteria suggested by Potter and Riessman may help to weed out weak research but are not intended to be absolute guarantees. What is important none the less is that attempts are made to conduct research in as scholarly a way as possible, to make appropriate claims about the strength of the findings, and to keep debating issues of validity and reliability in research.

Possible objections

The advantages of a research practice informed by postmodern feminist theory opens up new possibilities for undertaking research capable of handling complexity and continuing a commitment to social justice defined not just in terms of women, but men, women and children. Riessman's (1990) narrative research on violence in marriage is a case in point where the accounts of men and women are explored fully and in all their complexity unlike much of the standpoint theory-informed research on violence.

Yet the shift away from giving women a voice to identifying gendered narratives, from research on or with women to research on gender relations poses a real challenge to taken-for-granted assumptions about how research on gender should be done. One of the most challenging aspects is the stance taken towards the accounts given by research participants. Social work research on gender has traditionally emphasised building up trust and empathy with research participants and providing a platform for them to speak, generally taking what is said at face value. Peter Reason, who is strongly associated with participative research approaches, argues that poststructural approaches are nihilistic and oppressive, and that the first voices to be deconstructed are those of the oppressed, the poor and women (1994: 334). Indeed, it seems that by examining what discursive and rhetorical resources research participants are using we are being implicitly disrespectful, critical, or at best distrustful.

But equally there are dangers or risks if we fail to question how accounts are put together and how they seek to persuade. As Michelle Fine argues: 'This risk lies in the romanticizing of narratives and the concomitant retreat from analysis. In the name of ethical, democratic, sometimes feminist methods, there is a subtle, growing withdrawal from interpretation' (1994: 80–1). Researchers cannot presume, as standpoint theory suggests, that people act rationally in their own interests, that the oppressed can somehow stand outside of gender relations and do not have a will to power of their own. We cannot assume that women are always good and are to be believed, while men are always bad and to be distrusted. Instead, Fine argues postmodern feminist researchers should be 'Seeking to work with, but not romanticize, subjugated voices, searching for moments of social justice' (ibid.: 81). Postmodern feminism researchers therefore should be challenging rather than reproducing fixed gender categories in the interests of social justice, but this should be done explicitly, honestly and fairly.

Conclusion

This chapter has identified that most social work research does not address gender issues, while the standpoint feminist research which does so is in a way which remains wedded to fixed gender categories. A research practice informed by postmodern feminism as outlined above could make a major contribution to developing a body of research to inform social work practice in a way which does justice to the complexity of gendered social relations. Research on gender cannot just be about presenting women's voices, or presenting them in an unproblematic way.

I would not, however, argue that postmodern feminism research should be the only form of research which should be undertaken. There is some very good research on gender from a non-postmodern feminist standpoint but which attempts to do justice to the complexities of social life. Johnston and Campbell's (1993) development of a typology of a range of types of domestic violence is a case in point and of direct relevance to practice. Nor are all issues and questions which researchers might want to address able to be encapsulated by the types of research practice – narrative and discourse analysis – described above. As Filmer et al. (1998: 24–5) state, the world is not just a social construction. We still need to examine the gendered effects and outcomes of, say, child protection processes, as well as the processes and discourses which produce them. Thus a range of research methods are vital. The development of postmodern feminist theory as well as a research practice does however have much to contribute in its own right, as well as generating debate between researchers so that each makes theoretically informed decisions about what questions to ask and how to answer them.

Note

1   This section draws on the arguments developed more fully in Featherstone and Trinder (1997).

Bibliography

Bloom, M. (ed.) (1993) *Single-System Designs in the Social Services: Issues and Options for the 1990s*, New York: Haworth.

Bloom, M. and Block, S. (1977) 'Evaluating one's own effectiveness and efficiency', *Social Work* 22(2): 130–6.

Blythe, B. and Briar, S. (1985) 'Developing empirically based models of practice', *Social Work* 30(6): 483–8.

Cheetham, J., Fuller, R., McIvor, G. and Petch, A. (1992) *Evaluating Social Work Effectiveness*, Buckingham: Open University Press.

Coffey, A. and Atkinson, P. (1996) *Making Sense of Qualitative Data*, London: Sage.

Dartington Social Research Unit (1995) *Child Protection: Messages from Research*, London: HMSO.

Denzin, N. (1994) 'The art and politics of interpretation', in N. Denzin, and Y. Lincoln (eds) *Handbook of Qualitative Research*, Thousand Oaks, CA: Sage.

Denzin, N. and Lincoln, Y. (1994a) (eds) *Handbook of Qualitative Research*, Thousand Oaks, CA: Sage.

—— (1994b) 'Introduction', in N. Denzin, and Y. Lincoln (eds) *Handbook of Qualitative Research*, Thousand Oaks, CA: Sage.

Everitt, A. and Hardiker, P. (1996) *Evaluating for Good Practice*, Basingstoke: Macmillan.

Everitt, A., Hardiker, P., Littlewood, J. and Mullender, A. (1992) *Applied Research for Better Practice*, Basingstoke: Macmillan.

Featherstone, B. and Trinder, L. (1997) 'Familiar subjects? Domestic violence and child welfare', *Child and Family Social Work* 2(3): 147–59.

Filmer, P., Jenks, C., Seale, C., and Walsh, D. (1998) 'Developments in social theory', in C. Seale (ed.) *Researching Society and Culture*, London: Sage.

Fine, M. (1994) 'Working the hyphens', in N. Denzin and Y. Lincoln (eds) *Handbook of Qualitative Research*, Thousand Oaks, CA: Sage.

Fischer, J. (1973) 'Is casework effective?', *Social Work*, 1(5): 5–20.

—— (1976) *The Effectiveness of Social Casework*, Springfield, ILL: Charles C. Thomas.

Flax, J. (1990) *Thinking Fragments: Psychoanalysis, Feminism and Postmodernism in the Contemporary West*, Berkeley, CA: University of California Press.

—— (1993) *Disputed Subjects: Essays on Psychoanalysis, Politics and Philosophy*, London: Routledge.

Folkard, M.S., Smith, D.E. and Smith, D.D. (1976) *IMPACT: The Results of the Experiment*, Home Office Research Study Number 36, London: HMSO.

Fraser, N. (1989) 'Talking about needs: interpretative contests as political conflicts in welfare state societies', *Ethics*, 99(2): 291–313.

Fuller, R. (1996) 'Evaluating social work effectiveness: a pragmatic approach', in P. Alderson, S. Brill, I. Chalmers, R. Fuller, P. Hinkley-Smith, G. Macdonald, T. Newman, A. Oakley, H. Roberts and H. Ward (eds) *What Works? Effective Social Interventions in Child Welfare*, Ilford: Barnardos.

Fuller, R. and Petch, A. (1995) *Practitioner Research: The Reflexive Social Worker*, Buckingham: Open University Press.

Gill, R. (1996) 'Discourse analysis: practical implementation', in J. Richardson (ed.) *Handbook of Qualitative Research Methods for Psychology and the Social Sciences*, London: British Psychological Society.

Guba, E. and Lincoln, Y. (1994) 'Competing paradigms in qualitative research', in N. Denzin and Y. Lincoln (eds) *Handbook of Qualitative Research*, Thousand Oaks, CA: Sage.

Harding, S. (1991) *Whose Science? Whose Knowledge?*, Buckingham: Open University Press.

Hart, E. and Bond, M. (1995) *Action Research for Health and Social Care: A Guide to Practice*, Buckingham: Open University Press.

Hersen, M. and Barlow, D.H. (1976) *Single Case Experimental Designs: Strategies for Studying Behavior Change*, New York: Pergamon Press.

Hester, M. and Radford, L. (1996) *Domestic Violence and Child Contact Arrangements in England and Denmark*, Bristol: Policy Press.

Hollway, W. (1989) *Subjectivity and Method in Psychology: Gender, Meaning and Science*, London: Sage.

Home Office (1998) *Evidence-Based Practice: A Guide to Effective Practice*, London: Home Office.

Johnston, J. and Campbell, L. (1993) 'A clinical typology of interpersonal violence in disputed custody divorces', *American Journal of Orthopsychiatry* 63(2): 190–9.

Kelly, L. (1992) 'Journeying in reverse: possibilities and problems in feminist research on sexual violence', in L. Gelsthorpe and A. Morris (eds) *Feminist Perspectives in Criminology*, Milton Keynes: Open University Press.

Kelly, L., Regan, L. and Burton, S. (1991) *An Exploratory Study of the Prevalence of Sexual Abuse in a Sample of 1200 1—21 Year Olds*, Final Report submitted to ESRC, London: University of North London.

Lipton, D., Martinson, R. and Wilkes, J. (1975) *The Effectiveness of Correctional Treatment*, New York: Praeger.

Macdonald, G. (1996) 'Ice therapy: why we need randomised controlled trials', in P. Alderson, S. Brill, I. Chalmers, R. Fuller, P. Hinkley-Smith, G. Macdonald, T. Newman, A. Oakley, H. Roberts and H. Ward, *What Works? Effective Social Interventions in Child Welfare*, Barkingside: Barnardos.

—— (1997a) 'Social work: beyond control?', in A. Maynard, and I. Chalmers (eds) *Non-Random Reflections on Health Services Research*, London: BMJ.

—— (1997b) 'Social work research: the state we're in', *Journal of Interprofessional Care* 11(1): 57–65.

Macdonald, G. and Roberts, H. (1995) *What Works in the Early Years?*, Ilford: Barnardos.

Macdonald, G. and Sheldon, B. (1992) 'Contemporary studies of the effectiveness of social work', *British Journal of Social Work* 22(6): 614–43.

Martinson, R. (1974) 'What works? Questions and answers about prison reform', *Public Interest* 10(1): 405–17.

Mullen, E.J. and Dumpson, J.R. (1972) *Evaluation of Social Intervention*, San Francisco: Jossey-Bass.

NCH Action for Children (1994) *The Hidden Victims: Children and Domestic Violence*, London: National Children's Homes.

Potter, J. (1996) 'Discourse analysis and constructionist approaches: theoretical background', in J. Richardson (ed.) *Handbook of Qualitative Research Methods for Psychology and the Social Sciences*, London: British Psychological Society.

Potter, J. and Mulkay, M. (1985) 'Scientists' interview talk: interviews as a technique for revealing participants' interpretive practices', in M. Brenner, J. Brown and D. Canter (eds) *The Research Interview: Uses and Approaches*, London: Academic Press.

Potter, J. and Wetherell, M. (1995) 'Discourse analysis', in J. Smith, R. Harre, and K. Van Langenhove (eds) *Rethinking Methods in Psychology*, London: Sage.

Powers, E. and Witmer, H. (1951) *An Experiment in the Prevention of Delinquency: The Cambridge-Somerville Youth Study*, New York: Columbia University Press.

Reason, P. (1994) 'Three approaches to participative inquiry', in N. Denzin and Y. Lincoln (eds) *Handbook of Qualitative Research*, Thousand Oaks, CA: Sage.

Reid, W. and Hanrahan, P. (1980) 'The effectiveness of social work: recent evidence', in E. Goldberg and N. Connelly (eds) *Evaluative Research in Social Care*, London: Heinemann.

—— (1982) 'Recent evaluations of social work: grounds for optimism', *Social Work* 27(8): 328–40.

Riessman, C. (1990) *Divorce Talk: Men and Women Make Sense of Personal Relationships*, New Brunswick, NJ: Rutgers University Press.

—— (1993) *Narrative Analysis*, London: Sage.

—— (1994) 'Making sense of marital violence: one woman's narrative', in C. Riessman (ed.) *Qualitative Studies in Social Work Research*, London: Sage.

Rubin, A. (1985) 'Practice effectiveness: more grounds for optimism', *Social Work* 30: 469–76.

Sackett, D.L., Richardson, S., Rosenberg, W., and Haynes, R.B. (1997) *Evidence-Based Medicine: How to Practise and Teach EB*, London: Churchill-Livingstone.

Sackett, D.L., Rosenberg, W., Muir Gray, J., Haynes, R., Richardson, S. (1996) 'Evidence-based medicine: what it is and what it isn't', *British Medical Journal* 312(7023): 71–2.

Seale, C. (1998) 'Qualitative interviewing', in C. Seale (ed.) *Researching Society and Culture*, London: Sage.

Segal, S. (1972) 'Research on the outcomes of social work therapeutic interventions: a review of the literature', *Journal of Health and Social Behaviour* 13: 3–17.

Shaw, I. (1996) *Evaluating in Practice*, Aldershot: Arena.

Sheldon, B. (1983) 'The use of single case experimental designs in the evaluation of social work effectiveness', *British Journal of Social Work* 13(5): 477–500.

—— (1986) 'Social work effectiveness experiments: review and implications', *British Journal of Social Work* 16(2): 223–42.

Silverman, D. (1993) *Interpreting Qualitative Data*, London: Sage.

Smart, C. (1992) 'Feminist approaches to criminology or postmodern woman meets atavistic man', in L. Gelsthorpe and A. Morris (eds) *Feminist Perspectives in Criminology*, Buckingham: Open University Press.

Smith, D. (1987) 'The limits of positivism in social work research', *British Journal of Social Work* 17(4): 401–16.

Social Services Inspectorate (1995) *Domestic Violence and Social Care: A Report of Two Conferences held by the Social Services Inspectorate*, London: Department of Health.

Swigonski, M. (1993) 'Feminist standpoint theory and the questions of social work research', *Affilia* 8(2), Summer: 171–83.

Thomlinson, R. (1984) 'Something works: evidence from practice effectiveness studies', *Social Work* 29(2): 51–7.

Thyer, B. and Thyer, K. (1992) 'Single-system research designs in social work practice', *Research on Social Work Practice* 2(1): 99–116.

Tonkiss, F. (1998) 'Analysing discourse', in C. Seale (ed.) *Researching Society and Culture*, London: Sage.

Trinder, L. (1996) 'Social work research: the state of the art (or science)', *Child and Family Social Work* 1(4): 233–42.

—— (1999) 'Evidence-based social work', in S. Reynolds and L. Trinder (eds) *Evidence-Based Practice: A Critical Appraisal*, Oxford: Blackwell Science.

Tyson, K. (1995) *New Foundations for Scientific Social and Behavioural Research*, Boston: Allyn and Bacon.

Van Maanen, J. (1988) *Tales of the Field*, Chicago: University of Chicago Press.

Videka-Sherman, L. (1988) 'Meta-analysis of research on social work practice in mental health', *Social Work* 33(4): 325–38.

Witkin, S. (1996) 'If empirical practice is the answer, then what is the question?', *Social Work Research* 20(2): 69–75.

Wood, K.M. (1978) 'Casework effectiveness: a new look at the research evidence', *Social Work* 23(November): 437–59.

Chapter 4

Researching disability

Meanings, interpretations and analysis

Barbara Fawcett

Introduction

Theorising and researching are associated activities but the relationship between the two areas is often far from straightforward. This can be seen to be particularly the case when orientations drawn from postmodern feminism are applied to researching into 'disability'. The forging of appropriate links between postmodern feminist perspectives and empirical data and the devising of a workable analytical frame are two key areas which have to be addressed. These areas will be considered in this chapter, but first it is useful to highlight the reasons underpinning the undertaking of such research and to locate this project within the broader arena of social work.

The application of theory to practice within social work has been seen as a necessary, but complicated endeavour, finding favour more often with social work educators than with practitioners and managers. Social work is undergoing rationalisation and compartmentalisation and in many settings a managerial agenda which emphasises procedures takes precedence over critical analysis and informed reflection. This could be seen as part of the postmodern condition (Lyotard, 1994) if indeed, and this is a much disputed point, we could be seen to be living in a postmodern era. However, in relation to social work, performativity, which focuses on the carrying out of mandated tasks, is not enough. In the view of the author, there needs to be a concomitant emphasis on ideas, creativity, transferability and to use a word, much maligned by jargonistic usage, vision. In this scenario, the exploration of associations and tensions between theory and practice takes on another meaning, one which is both dynamic and challenging and, it is contended, important to the continuation of social work, as a multifaceted, critically reflective and productive activity.

The research project discussed in this chapter can be seen as an attempt to make connections between theory and research practice. It does not seek to be prescriptive, nor to participate in the formulation of a definitive model, rather, the purpose is to generate ideas and debate, facilitate further connections and to take part in the process outlined above. A starting point for this endeavour will be a brief discussion about how terms such as 'disability' and 'postmodern feminism' are being used. Links between theoretical perspectives and research methodology will then be discussed and examples will be given of this particular version of researching into 'disability' using postmodern feminist perspectives. Finally, the applicability of perspectives emanating from postmodern feminism to both the arena of disability and the field of social work will be considered.

'Disability': a contested area

'Disability' can be regarded as a contested area. Views of what constitute 'normality' and abnormality are influenced at both macro and micro levels by cultural and social factors, physical environments and by historical location. All language used in the context of 'disability' can be seen to be tainted and issues of representation are fraught with difficulty to the extent that how 'disability' is represented and by whom, can be seen to affect conceptualisations and recommended outcomes (G. Williams, 1996). Attempts to define 'disability' raise ontological, epistemological, political and moral issues and as Wendell asserts: 'Questions of definition arise in countless practical situations, influence social policies and determine outcomes that profoundly affect the lives of people with disabilities' (1996: 11).

In recent years debates have centred on two 'models' of disability – the social model of disability and its refuted binary opposite – the 'individual' or medical model of disability. By reference to the social model of disability, the medical model of disability places emphasis on individual impairments and classification systems. If an impairment cannot be 'cured', then the only humane alternative is 'care' and the subjecting of individuals to 'care and control' regimes (Finkelstein, 1993). Individuals with impairments are either encouraged to become passively dependent, or exhorted to strive towards 'independence', even if the completion of personal tasks constitutes an energy-draining and time-consuming process. Autonomy, or the full involvement of the disabled person in making decisions about all aspects of their life, tend not to feature as key areas warranting attention. In psychological terms, individuals are counselled to come to terms with their position and to adjust to the loss of normality, with conversely, 'normality' also being cited as the goal to which they should continually strive.

If the medical model of disability can be seen to be based on methodological individualism, which has as its adjunct, psychologically orientated explanations of how an individual can adjust to their impairment (Shakespeare, 1994), the social model of disability in contrast highlights a materialist structuralist approach. The social model focuses on the effects of personal and institutionalised prejudice. 'Disability' is not an individual issue, but is created by environmental and social factors. It is external restraints which disable, not individual impairments. Disability Rights Campaigns based on the social model of disability make it clear that disablism is further perpetuated at individual and institutional levels by a general lack of access to public places and transport and that despite the passing of ameliorative legislation (e.g. in Britain the Disability Discrimination Act 1995), there remains much to be done in terms of the acquisition of full social, political and economic rights associated with citizenship.

At this point it has to be stated that the understanding of 'disability' used both in this chapter and for the purposes of the research project has been strongly influenced by the social model of disability. However, the influence of this model is not straightforward. On the one hand, it is accepted that the political significance of the social model of disability has been considerable. It has undoubtedly facilitated positive and constructive challenges to previously dominant conceptualisations of disability and disabling images and has generated a re-appraisal of social work services to disabled individuals. On the other, problem areas, related to the exploration of difference and diversity associated with dimensions such as gender, 'race', age, class and impairment, remain. Discussion relating to whether differences between disabled people ought to be explored (e.g. Begum, 1992; Morris, 1993, 1996; Crow, 1996), or whether such explorations ought to be avoided or sidelined, on the basis that they could adversely affect the projected unity of disability rights movements and the associated political impact, are currently taking place between supporters of the social model. French (1993) for example, accepts that placing emphasis on difference is potentially problematic but argues that difference and diversity between and amongst disabled people has to be explored even if this does stretch the boundaries of an extremely useful model. This view is shared by the author, although in line with orientations emanating from postmodern feminism, explanations of difference based on essentialistic notions of experience advocated by writers such as Begum, (1992); French (1993), Morris (1993, 1996) and Crow (1996) are eschewed.

Postmodern feminism

With regard to the research project, a key focus has related to how subjects are constructed, for example, in relation to the conceptualisations of 'disability' operating and also how subjects are able to construct and critique. Foucault (1979, 1981a, 1981b, 1986) and Derrida (1978), both influential in the formulation of poststructural and postmodern perspectives,[1] tend to view subjects as effects of discourse or as positions in language. Many feminists would agree with Benhabib (1995) who maintains that postmodern and poststructural concepts of subjectivity, which reject liberal views of the 'individual' as essentially unified, coherent and rational, are not compatible with feminist politics. However, by utilising the work of authors who have engaged with postmodernism and feminism, it is possible to present a version of postmodern feminism which rejects humanistic conceptions of self, yet moves away from merely seeing the subject as constructed by discourse. Consequently a form of agency remains possible. The contribution of these perspectives will now be briefly explored.

Weedon regards subjects as both the 'site and subjects of discursive struggle for their identity' (1987: 97). In terms of subjectivity and the social, identities are regarded as multiple and subjectivity, as precarious and contradictory. However, the position of a subject within discourse is always open to challenge, and is never final. There is also always room for resistance. Moore (1994) maintains that subjectivity is non-unitary and multiple. She regards subjectivity as the product of variable discourses and practices, but does not deny agency. Focusing on gender differences she asserts that: 'women and men come to have different understandings of themselves as engendered persons because they are differentially positioned with regard to discourses concerning gender and sexuality and they take up different positions within those discourses' (Moore, 1994: 64).

Flax (1992) constructively critiques understandings of both modern or Enlightenment perspectives of 'self' and also postmodern positionings of 'self'. With regard to modern orientations, Flax rejects universalistic and essentialist underpinnings and argues that a feminist view of an interconnected, integrated and social 'self' differs from the Enlightenment view of 'self' where individuality is regarded as unique and based on essentialist and rational features. In terms of postmodern formulations, she rejects concepts of 'self' which deny agency. Flax maintains that a postmodern feminist 'self' would have to be non-objective, non-rational and historically grounded. It would also have to be differentiated and local, but it could, she contends, be a social 'self' (Flax, 1992: 201; Fawcett and Featherstone, 1998).

Butler (1995) argues that contentions such as those made by Benhabib (1995), that postmodern conceptions of subjectivity are incompatible with feminism, are based on a foundationalist premise, the deconstruction of which, rather than being destructive for feminism, could be regarded as constructive. According to Butler, the notion of agency can be reconceptualised so that it is not either assumed or rejected as a given, but is related to the exploration of particular conditions which may render 'mobilisation' possible (1995: 47). In other words the subject is both constructed through mechanisms of power and exclusions, but in certain contexts there are opportunities for resignification and action. Butler (1995) maintains that 'agency' is facilitated if fixed referents are eschewed. She argues, for example, that by paradoxically freeing 'woman' from a fixed categorical referent related to identity, 'agency' becomes possible in that if referents are not fixed, then a wide range of new configurations are produced. She states that if 'woman' is used to 'designate an undesignatable field of differences, one that cannot be totalized or summarized by a descriptive identity category, then the very term becomes a site of permanent openness and resignifiability' (Butler, 1995: 50).

The authors discussed above all arrive at different conceptualisations and indeed there can be clear points of disagreement. Fraser (1995), for example, makes a contribution which takes issue with Butler's use of esoteric language and maintains that 'resignification' is used in her discourse as she uses 'critique' in hers. However, 'critique' carries with it connotations of justification and warrant and consequently 'critique' can be presented as positive whereas 'resignification' is merely neutral. Fraser (1995) argues for new paradigms of feminist theorising which integrate, rather than polarise the insights of Critical Theory with the insights of postmodernism.

Overall, taking on board variations and disagreements, it can be argued that perspectives emanating from postmodern feminism facilitate the reintroduction of notions of 'self' and subjectivity in ways that do not privilege experience, but which decentre subjects, point to non-essentialist features which are always in process and which regard the 'self' or subject as a predominantly social entity. Subjects are not regarded as merely occupying discursive positions, but can be seen as both constructed or positioned and capable of construction, or positioning and critique.

Considerable attention has been paid to this aspect of postmodern feminism because it relates so directly to a key aspect of the methodological frame used in this research project. However, before moving on to explore methodological issues in greater detail, it is useful to briefly explore similarities and differences between postmodernism and postmodern feminism. This endeavour will also highlight other facets of postmodern feminism which have influenced the research project.

Postmodern approaches reject the persuasive power of grand narratives, the view that certainty is ever obtainable and the existence of an essentialist foundation for individual identity and social structure. Key aspects of postmodern orientations can be seen to be: pluralism and a concomitant emphasis on difference, diversity, fluidity and change; relativism, which incorporates an acceptance that 'objective' knowledge, the 'truth' of any situation and the rational underpinnings that provide a power/knowledge basis for mastery (Docherty, 1993) are impossible to achieve; and fragmentation, in that unifying coherent bases for knowledge claims and political action are rendered unacceptable. Postmodern perspectives also dismiss essentialist notions of experience and accept the non-viability of ahistorical metanarratives and the notion of a subject of history.

Postmodern applications can be seen to have resulted in deconstructive criticisms of rationality, binary pairings, the operation of modernist power/knowledge frameworks and essentialist and foundationalist dogma. However, there are problem areas, particularly in relation to relativity and the impossibility of weighting one claim against another. These aspects have brought into question the utility of postmodern conceptualisations for those who want to retain access to the critically analytical, yet socially located strengths of feminism. However, the argument presented here is that by engaging with writers who have sought (in varying ways) to embrace postmodern feminism, it is possible to present reformulations. Accordingly, it can be contended that postmodern feminism, in relation to power/knowledge frameworks, emphasises historical location and the ability to weight sites of contestation both contextually and intercontextually. With regard to notions of subjectivity and views of 'self', social aspects and the ways in which different 'identities' can be utilised in a number of contexts are highlighted. Subjects are not regarded as merely being positioned by the various discourses operating, but are seen as both constructed and capable of construction and critique. In relation to matters of difference, there is an emphasis on viewing it as a resource rather than as an obstacle. With regard to political change, the potential to re-invigorate non-essentialist forms of representational politics based on a temporary freezing of differences, is emphasised (F. Williams, 1996). The notion of 'identity politics' is also eschewed in favour of strategic alliances which emphasise connectedness and inclusiveness, rather than marginality and exclusive differentness. These areas will be explored more fully later in the chapter when the applicability of postmodern feminism to the disability arena and to social work will be examined. However, it is important to re-emphasise here that orientations emanating from postmodern feminism can be seen as having a contribution to make to researching and practising in the related areas of disability and social work.

The deconstructive textual analysis: some considerations

The perspectives derived from postmodern feminism discussed above have informed the research project which has concentrated on a deconstructive textual analysis of twenty-five accounts read as texts given by people (fourteen women and eleven men)[2] who were drawn from four different settings. These settings comprised an 'innovative' residential centre, where operating practices were informed by the social model of disability, a 'traditional' residential centre, where a number of residents at the time the interviews took place were being required to move into the community, a day centre and the community. The accounts were generated by means of an interview format, which initially used a general prompt to enable the respondents to create their own narrative and generate their own order which could then be seen to make sense sequentially and holistically. To illustrate, all the respondents were initially asked: 'Can you tell me what you understand by "disability"' / 'What does disability mean to you?'.[3] The intention was for the interviews to: 'generate their own coherence through their responsiveness to the concerns of the participant' (Opie, 1992: 57). All interviews were taped and fully transcribed.

At a methodological level, perspectives emanating from postmodern feminism have informed the research project in that what is said and the positions displayed in the context of the research study have been regarded as being constructed in particular settings and laid down as texts. Interview responses have not been seen as giving rise to essentialist or uniquely privileged accounts that discover 'the truth' of a situation, but as capturing meanings that are context-specific and bound up with the varying discursive practices operating. Meanings have also been regarded as being continually created and re-created in language, and there is an acceptance that meanings can be fixed or frozen for a finite period and used as the basis for study. As highlighted above, particular emphasis has been placed not only on how a subject is positioned in the text, but also upon how they in turn position themselves and utilise the discursive or cultural or ideological resources at their disposal. Specific analytical tools have also been developed to facilitate this interpretative process. These tools include the paying of attention to the styles, emotional tones and intensities used within the texts (Opie, 1992) and the noting of variations, contradictions and paradox (Potter and Wetherell, 1987, 1994; Billig 1987; Burman and Parker 1993; Widdicombe 1993 and Macnaghten 1993). Interpretative shifts, which relate to the ways in which the subject develops the account or interprets prompts are also highlighted, as are omissions or gaps. With regard to this latter area, Opie (1992) asserts that omissions and what is not said have the potential to be as revealing as that which is said and included in the text.

Deconstructive textual analysis: an application

In this chapter, both in relation to the discussion of postmodern feminist perspectives and with regard to the methodological framework, a central linking tenet has been how subjects can be regarded as being both positioned in discourse (or constructed) and also capable of negotiating discursive positions (or constructing and critiquing). The application of this positioning and the use made of the analytical tools will now be explored further by focusing on the analysis of two texts from two of the case study settings, the 'innovative' residential centre and the traditional residential centre.

The text of S from the 'innovative' residential centre can be seen to be particularly interesting with regard to omissions in that 'disability' is not mentioned at all. In relation to the opening question about what 'disability' means to the respondent, S immediately asks if the interviewer is married. In the text, she continually ignores prompts about disability and politely asks repetitive questions about the researcher's own family and talks about her own. However, S's family are absent and although in the text 'going home' is an area continually referred to, at the time of the interview, staff at the centre pointed out that her husband has divorced her. She also rarely sees her grown-up son and daughter, both of whom live a considerable distance away and have families of their own. It is possible that for S, 'disability' is about the loss of her family. It is also possible that she does not want to talk about 'disability' for emotional reasons, or perhaps her impairment (Multiple Sclerosis) has affected her mental capacity to the extent that her communicative abilities have been reduced to a formulaic pattern. Another reading is that although her family are not with her, by talking about them, S appears not so much to feel their loss, but to re-create their presence and to remould them in images which are comforting and acceptable to her. By having a family, she also has a point of contact with others and is able to focus on sameness rather than difference and to retain a means of communication, when other, more complicated means are perhaps not available to her. In the text alternative stances do not feature for S, or are ignored. One reading is that she has produced her own script and refuses to deviate from it.

With regard to how S is positioned in relation to 'disability' and constructions associated with the 'medical model' and the social model, she could be positioned within a 'medical model' frame by the social model of disability, with emphasis being placed on the avoidance of disability and upon striving for approximations of 'normality'. However, overall, it is S's own positioning or construction which appears to dominate. It also has to be emphasised that this construction is very social, and interactive. She could also be seen to adopt a gendered subject position in terms of the prominent place she affords to her family in the text.

In contrast to S, A and J, a married couple from the traditional residential centre, both clearly regard themselves as 'disabled'. The style adopted in this text is predominantly descriptive and displays a desire on the part of both to be as helpful as possible. However, levels of emotional intensity vary at particular points in the text. J for example, becomes emotional when talking about her parents, her father's death and her fears about having to move into the community, which both may be 'required' to do. A is much quieter than J and tends to leave J to do most of the talking, although he listens carefully and intervenes quickly when she becomes upset. His measured tone changes only at the prospect of a move into the community and when talking about his mother, to whom he was very close and the attitude of an aunt who lives nearby and who did not come to their wedding.

Variations, contradictions and paradox particularly feature in the text in relation to the discussion about 'care' and the possibility of a move into the community. Both A and J regard 'disability' as requiring both emotional and physical 'care' and they use 'care' to denote both aspects. This is what they have received and it forms part of their continued expectations. However, there are some discordant notes in the text in relation to 'care'. J for example appreciates that she needs help, particularly when climbing stairs, yet she also feels that 'care' staff are overprotective and that she is being constrained by their helpfulness. J also wants 'care' staff to be available when she needs them – for a bath, for example – and is critical of staff not being able to assist at times of need. However, later in the text, when the discussion has shifted to the possibility of A and J having to move out into the community, she makes light of the demands she places on 'care' staff because she feels they are more likely to be allowed to stay, rather than be obliged to move into the community if they are regarded as undemanding residents. With regard to paradox, A and J maintain repeatedly in the text that they feel fully involved in the changes taking place at the centre and stress the fact that they are on the committee. However, they also allude throughout the text to the strong possibility that they will be required, against their better judgement, to move into the community. If this happens they feel they will have no option, but to get on with it. In the text, they do not see themselves as occupying contradictory positions.

When looking at how A and J position themselves in relation to disability, it is apparent that for them, their construction of disability has been positive. They have received a lot of 'care' and project positive self-images – the unhappiness they have experienced has either been caused through the death of a parent, or through the interventions of 'others', in terms of recommended courses of action and enforced change. An interesting interpretative shift in relation to this latter point occurs in that discussion about J's education is dominated by her experience of being assessed and sent away, against her wishes, from her parents to a boarding school. A textual reading of this situation highlights the potential irony of a child being sent away from her parents who live in the community, to boarding school in order to obtain a 'normalising' experience aimed at equipping her as far as possible to live in the community.

In the text, the support which A and J obtain from each other is highlighted and it is clear that they enjoy a form of autonomy greater than each would have on their own. However, they feel they need a parental figure to look out for them and this is the role played by the centre. The community 'out there' is viewed as unfriendly, unsupportive and possibly dangerous. Notions of autonomy and rights are meaningless terms for A and J. However, this enhances their vulnerability in that if the centre changes, they do not have the personal resources to try to ensure that their expressed needs are met. There is also the paradox that they have come to expect professional 'others' to make decisions for them, decisions which they may regard with anxiety and apprehension, yet both appear to need and want professional 'others' to continue to occupy a parental role.

A and J can be seen to share many subject positions in that they both position themselves as requiring 'care' and they also position themselves as being wary of professional assessments and the consequences of these. However, A and J can also be seen to occupy subject positions which the other does not share. J, for example, in the text tends to focus on what she cannot do and talks about her body in terms of its unpredictability. A does not focus on difficulties experienced through his visual impairment at all (with the exception of how he is limited by the weather). He positions himself in terms of what he can do, rather than what he cannot, stressing abilities rather than dis-abilities. This could be regarded as a gendered construction. It is interesting to note that this positioning marks a variation to the way A and J generally construct themselves in the text as a mutually complementary couple who resist gendered subject positions. A reading of this construction could be that their adult/child relationship with the centre frees them from the gendered constraints placed on other married couples. The fact that both entered residential care from family situations relatively recently also suggests that they may not have been subject to the same gendered 'normalising' approaches as others who have spent longer periods in similar establishments. This reading is also supported by an omission in the text relating to children. Neither A nor J refer to having children and this may reflect the way they see themselves – as individuals in need of parental support, or in line with a paternalistic and paternalising discourse, may relate to the ways in which they have learnt to perceive themselves as incapable of looking after children.

With regard to the social model of disability, both A and J could be positioned as being subject to 'false consciousness' in that their view of their situation, lacking an analysis drawn from the social model of disability does not take into account disabling forces and the need for challenge and change. In relation to this latter point, they could be constructed as victims of a 'care and control' culture. The social model would construct them as having a limited number of positions to occupy. The position they do occupy could be seen to be that of 'professional cripples' (Shakespeare, 1996) and they could be constructed as having accepted external disempowering constructions. In this context, it is interesting to speculate whether an emphasis on rights and autonomy (social model) by either J's family or professionals or both, would have led to her not going to boarding school and whether not going, would have changed her discursive positioning.

The purpose of including these analytic extracts has been both to illustrate how a deconstructive textual analysis could be conducted and also to make links between theory and practice, which in the context of this chapter has been postmodern feminism and research practice. With regard to the deconstructive textual analysis, the style or styles used, the emotional tones and intensities, the omissions, variations, contradictions, paradoxes and interpretative shifts found in the text have all been highlighted with the purpose of breaking down the text and paying particular attention to detail. Emphasis has also been placed on how subjects are both constructed or positioned and construct or position (and also critique). The impact of the social and medical models of disability, with regard to the positions occupied, has also been appraised.

Deconstructive readings can be seen to present 'disability' as impacting in a variety of ways on individuals at differing textual junctures. It is contended that the application of perspectives drawn from postmodern feminism facilitates a form of textual analysis which 'hears' the differing voices and proffers readings which always contain the possibility of alternatives. In such readings discursive positionings feature, but agency is still possible and emphasis is placed on multiple constructions and upon variation.

The application of reformulations drawn from postmodern feminism to disability and social work

At this point, it is pertinent to review how orientations emanating from postmodern feminism can be seen to have relevance for debates in relation to both disability and social work. Shakespeare and Watson (1997) maintain that it is both possible and desirable to retain the social model of disability within a more nuanced worldview drawing from feminist and postmodern accounts.[4] This can be seen to be a theoretically general and somewhat optimistic stance in that Fawcett (1996) argues that it is ironic that just as disability rights campaigns based on the social model of disability have finally achieved political and social prominence in Britain and internationally, their structuralist foundations are challenged by poststructural and postmodern orientations. From a postmodern perspective, modernist notions of rights and citizenship can be seen to give way to an emphasis on relativity, pluralism and provisionality. However, perspectives emanating from postmodern feminism can be seen to allow for the recognition of rights. Foundationally orientated universal notions of rights linked to metanarratives are rejected, but specific conceptualisations of rights, closely linked to specific pieces of legislation and contextually located are utilisable.

In addition, with regard to notions of citizenship, Flax's (1992) reformulated conceptualisation which links citizenship to a form of justice focusing on the reconciliation of diversities, reciprocity, recognition and judgement (viewed as a sense of balancing and proportion), can be seen to have something to offer. Flax stresses interconnectedness and mutual dependence, as well as separateness and distinctiveness and also maintains that 'there is nothing outside our tissue of practices, our mutually created transitional spaces, that can help us make decisions and relate to each other justly within them' (ibid.: 207). According to Flax, a move away from structural, religious or objective underpinnings for justice and citizenship, increases responsibility, both individually, in relation to changing conceptions of self and also collectively. Flax maintains that there is much to be gained by the collapse of the 'longest lie' (ibid.: 207, drawing on Nietzsche) and the recognition that justice is 'dependent solely upon our fragile and unstable selves' (ibid.: 208). In relation to disability movements based on the social model of disability, this perspective obviates the need to justify the fight for rights. All are involved and all are interconnected with regard to citizenship and justice.

Rattansi (1995), in the context of a discussion of ethnicities and racisms in a postmodern framework also points out that the notion of a 'self' that is always in process, the occupation of varying subject positions and a discursively constituted sense of identity, can result in particular discourses, particularly those relating to fairness and justice, being more attractive. Although there are dangers of fragmentation, the 'pull' of such discourses includes the potential 'for the mobilisation of otherwise disparately located subjects by movements struggling for anti-discriminatory and redistributive reform' (Rattansi, 1995: 279).

Such mobilisation could impact on disability rights movements in ways which avoid marginalisation, foster coalitions, recognise diversity and facilitate a move away from the projected homogeneity of disability rights campaigns based on the social model of disability. In relation to the latter, comparisons can be made with how the utility of 'Black' as a unifying signifier in the creation of a positive image has been losing its unifying effectiveness in ethnic minority politics. As Rattansi (1995) points out, the politics of representation (which has drawn attention to the huge variety of 'identities' present in minority communities) together with experimentation with postmodernist forms, has facilitated a break with the stifling aesthetic of 'realism' imposed by the demands of the 'positive' image. Accordingly, new forms of non-essentialist 'identity' formation, which highlight variety, mutuality and interconnectedness, as well as difference and diversity and which foster the interplay of ablebodiedness and disabledbodiedness, professionalism, non-professionalism, gender, sexualities, culture, subcultures, and so on, can be explored without losing sight of political issues.

With regard to power/knowledge frameworks, drawing on postmodern feminism, the reformulation(s) proposed facilitate a move away from taken-for-granted assumptions and accepted conceptual frameworks. Medical models are explored in the context of other models and the dangers of the social model being seen to constitute privileged knowledge is also highlighted. Any approach, no matter how liberatory and challenging it first appears, has the potential to become inflexible and rigid. Accordingly, the importance of subjecting such approaches to ongoing deconstructive appraisal is emphasised, as is the importance of paying attention to practices and contexts.

Orientations derived from postmodern feminism also draw attention to the utility of exploring paradox and contradiction. These can be seen to be aspects so often smoothed over or ignored in modern or structural accounts, where consistency and rational linear progression are insisted upon. The utility of the examination of paradox in relation to the research project can be highlighted by focusing on an area of omission that concerns 'the body'. Wendell (1996) maintains that attempting to disengage oneself from the body by ignoring its needs is generally a luxury of the healthy and ablebodied. She asserts that for disabled people, a fairly high degree of attention to the body is necessary both for survival and for preventing physical deterioration.

In relation to the research project, the lack of a focus on the body by the subjects can be regarded as a significant omission. One reading is perhaps that in order to survive, an individual who requires a considerable amount of physical assistance and who is used to being handled, places distance between their sense of 'self' and what is happening to their body. In many of the texts, discussions about 'their' body is subsumed into a discussion about disability and a further reading is that talking about 'their' bodies is an area which has not been encouraged, or has possibly even been discouraged. As a result bodies, bodily functions and the management of these are areas which are often given indirect (e.g. emphasis placed on toilet breaks) rather than direct expression.

Perspectives emanating from postmodern feminism also facilitate deconstructive, yet located appraisals. Fawcett and Featherstone (1998) argue that areas such as quality assurance and evaluation (viewed as objective, rational tools of efficiency and effectiveness), when applied to the field of disability, social work and health can be seen to form part of a modernist project applied to a postmodern era, where the large certainties of modernism have been shrivelled to 'small certainties'.[5] In relation to professional responses to disabled individuals, emphasis on 'small certainties' can be seen to result in the placing of a disproportionate emphasis on features such as assessment, monitoring, evaluation and particular management strategies which are regarded as all-defining and all-pervasive. Such a reliance on 'small certainties' can be seen to run counter to claims by disabled service users, based on the social model of disability, for autonomy, control, self assessment and rights (Fawcett and Featherstone, 1998). The binary reliance on 'small absolutes' can be seen to result in the paradox whereby the use of modernist 'small certainties' by professionals working with those categorised as disabled, can be viewed as counterproductive by disabled service users, whose arguments for change are also located within modernist structuralist perspectives (Fawcett, 1996).

The reformation(s) propounded also lead to a rejection of the modernist view of 'professionals' as 'experts' who in a rational and logical manner objectively assess, plan and determine outcomes. The perpetration of either/or scenarios where the rights and needs of disabled people are set up in binary opposition to the rights and needs of ablebodied people are similarly dismissed. Claims that there are unified, undifferentiated categorised groupings occupying positions on either side of a continuum can be deconstructed and seen as unjustifiable and counterproductive. Accordingly, there is an emphasis on negotiation in specific contexts with neither the perspectives of the service user(s) nor the professional(s)/agency(ies) being uniquely privileged, but with the weighting of specific claims remaining a contextual possibility. An example that can be used here is that of A and J from Case Study Two. A and J want to stay in their current establishment, yet the Social Services Department may require them to move out. The acceptance that neither claim is uniquely privileged results in the imposition of one perspective becoming unjustifiable. There is a need to negotiate. If a move is inevitable because of the impossibility of the establishment meeting new standards, A and J could insist on moving to a facility where they not only have autonomy, but access to 24-hour 'care' as required.

Perspectives drawn from postmodern feminism deconstruct accept power/knowledge frameworks, yet retain the ability to weight criteria in specific contexts; they highlight the variations offered by the notion of changing subjectivities, but also emphasise social and interrelated aspects and positively explore difference and diversity, while recognising and responding to social divisions. With regard to the arena of disability, these perspectives can be seen to foster an 'inclusive' rather than an 'exclusive' emphasis. Accordingly, exclusive, privileged positions, prescriptions and solutions are rejected. Instead there is an emphasis on inclusive features relating to notions of 'self', identity, experience and group alignments being viewed as in process and open to re-interpretation, with temporary agreements and courses of action being based on recognition and collaboration.

Concluding remarks

In terms of the discursive practices operating with regard to disability, that of absence predominates (Hearn, 1999).[6] Disabled people are ignored or regarded as a marginalised 'other' and ablebodiedness is assumed in a non-problematic manner. The textual readings discussed in this chapter have focused on disability, as presence, rather than absence, but they are the textual readings of a female researcher who is not 'registered disabled' and this has to be borne in mind when the various readings are considered.

As mentioned in the introduction, there are many ways of linking theoretical material to both researching and practising within the broad arena of both disability and social work. The associations discussed here are not intended to be prescriptive, rather, the intention has been to explore how orientations emanating from postmodern feminism can be used to research into 'disability' and to make links between theory and practice in ways which are simultaneously utilisable, theoretically challenging and practically applicable.

Notes

1 In this chapter, 'postmodern' incorporates poststructural perspectives (see Chapter 1).
2 Four of the respondents came from Black and Asian communities. The small number of Black and Asian respondents included in the study reflects the ethnic composition of the settings utilised.
3 Additional areas, relating to how respondents viewed themselves in relation to their understandings of 'disability' and how they regarded the attitudes of non-disabled people towards them were introduced by means of checklist prompts. The use of a checklist ensured that particular areas were covered without interfering with the narrative styles of the respondents. A number of respondents, without further prompting, went on to talk about all of the areas covered by the checklist prompts. When a respondent did not raise a particular area, a prompt related to this research question was used at an appropriate juncture in the narrative. Similarly, where respondents did not develop a narrative style, the prompts were used to promote discussion and generate the account.
4 Shakespeare and Watson (1997) do not appear to closely examine the opportunities and constraints posed by postmodernism for the social model of disability. They also do not appear to make links and explore tensions between feminism, postmodernism and postmodern feminism.
5 It is acknowledged that there is considerable debate as to whether we are living in a postmodern era (e.g. Bauman, 1992; Howe, 1994) and what the effects of postmodernity are.
6 Hearn's (1999) discursive analysis refers to men and masculinities.

Bibliography

Barrett, M. (1992) 'Words and things: materialism and method in contemporary feminist analysis', in M. Barrett and A. Phillips (eds) *Destabilising Theory: Contemporary Feminist Debates*, Cambridge: Polity Press.

Barton, L. and Oliver, M. (eds) (1996) *Disability Studies: Past Present and Future*, Leeds: The Disability Press.

Bauman, Z. (1992) *Intimations of Postmodernity*, London: Routledge.

Begum, N. (1992) 'Disabled women and the feminist agenda', *Feminist Review*, 40(42): 70–84.

Benhabib, S. (1995) 'Feminism and postmodernism', in *Feminist Contentions: A Philosophical Exchange*, London: Routledge.

Best, S. and Kellner, D. (1991) *Postmodern Theory: Critical Interrogations*, Basingstoke: Macmillan.

Billig, M. (1987) *Arguing and Thinking: A Rhetorical Approach to Social Psychology*, Cambridge: Cambridge University Press.

Burman, E. and Parker, I. (1993) (eds) *Discourse Analytic Research*, London: Routledge.

Butler, J. (1993) Bodies That Matter: On the Discursive Limits of 'Sex', London: Routledge.

—— (1995) 'Contingent foundations', in L. Nicholson (ed.) *Feminist Contentions: A Philosophical Exchange*, London: Routledge.

Crow, L. (1996) 'Including all of our lives: renewing the social model of disability', in C. Barnes and G. Mercer (eds) *Exploring the Divide: Illness and Disability*, Leeds: The Disability Press.

Derrida, J. (1978) *Writing and Difference*, trans. A Bass, Chicago: University of Chicago Press.

Docherty, M. (1993) *Postmodernism: A Reader*, Hemel Hempstead: Harvester Wheatsheaf.

Fawcett, B. (1996) 'Postmodernism, feminism and disability', *Scandinavian Journal of Social Welfare*, 14(3): 259–67.

—— (1998) 'Disability and social work: applications from poststructuralism, postmodernism and feminism', *British Journal of Social Work* 28: 263–77.

Fawcett, B. and Featherstone, B. (1997) 'Postmodernism, feminism and social work', *Social Work Review, (New Zealand)* March/June, IX(1 and 2): 3–9.

—— (1998) 'Quality assurance and evaluation in social work in a postmodern era', in J. Carter (ed.) *Postmodernity and the Fragmentation of Welfare*, London: Routledge.

Finkelstein, V. (1993) 'Disability: an administrative challenge? (The health and welfare heritage)', in M. Oliver (ed.) *Social Work: Disabled People and Disabling Environments*, Research Highlights in Social Work 2, London: Jessica Kingsley.

Flax, J. (1992) 'Beyond equality, gender, justice and difference', in L. Bock and S. James (eds) *Beyond Equality and Difference*, London: Routledge.

Foucault, M. (1979) *Discipline and Punish*, Harmondsworth: Penguin.

—— (1980) 'Body/Power', in C. Gordon (ed.) *Michel Foucault: Power/Knowledge: Selected Interviews and Other Writings 1972–1977*, Hemel Hempstead: Harvester Wheatsheaf.

—— (1981a) *The History of Sexuality, Volume One, An Introduction*, Harmondsworth: Pelican.

—— (1981b) 'Question of method: an interview with Michel Foucault', *Ideology and Consciousness* 8: 1–14.

—— (1986) *The History of Sexuality, Volume Two, The Use of Pleasure,* Harmondsworth: Viking.

Fraser, N. (1993) *Unruly Practices: Power, Discourse and Gender in Contemporary Social Theory,* Cambridge: Polity Press.

—— (1995) 'False antithesis', in L. Nicholson (ed.) *Feminist Contentions: A Philosophical Exchange,* London: Routledge.

Fraser, N. and Nicholson, L. (1993) 'Social criticism without philosophy: an encounter between feminism and postmodernism', in M. Docherty (ed) *Postmodernism: A Reader,* Hemel Hempstead: Harvester Wheatsheaf.

French, S. (1993) 'Disability, impairment or something in between?', in J. Swain, V. Finkelstein, S. French and M. Oliver (eds) *Disabling Barriers – Enabling Environments,* London: Sage.

Hearn, J. (1999) 'Theorising men and men's theorising: varieties of discursive practices in men's theorising of men', *Theory and Society* 27(6):781–816.

Howe, D. (1994) 'Surface and depth in social work practice', in N. Parton (ed.) *Social Theory, Social Change and Social Work,* London: Routledge.

Lyotard, J.F. (1994) *The Postmodern Condition: A Report on Knowledge,* Manchester: Manchester University Press (original 1984).

Macnaghten, P. (1993) 'Discourses of nature: argumentation and power', in E. Burman and I. Parker (eds) *Discourse Analytic Research,* London: Sage.

Moore, H.L. (1994) *A Passion for Difference,* Cambridge: Polity Press.

Morris, J. (1993) *Pride Against Prejudice,* London: Women's Press.

—— (ed.) (1996) *Encounters with Strangers: Feminism and Disability,* London: Women's Press.

Oliver, M. (1996) *Understanding Disability: From Theory to Practice,* Basingstoke: Macmillan.

Opie, A. (1992) 'Qualitative research, appropriation of the 'other' and empowerment', *Feminist Review* 40–2: 52–69.

Potter, J. and Wetherell, M. (1987) *Discourse and Social Psychology,* London: Sage.

—— (1994) 'Analysing discourse', in A. Bryman and R.G. Burgess (eds) *Analysing Qualitative Data,* London: Routledge.

Rattansi, A. (1995) 'Just framing: ethnicities and racisms in a "postmodern" framework', in L. Nicholson and S. Seidman (eds) *Social Postmodernism: Beyond Identity Politics,* Cambridge: Cambridge University Press.

Sarup, M. (1993) *Poststructuralism and Postmodernism,* Hemel Hempstead: Harvester Wheatsheaf.

Shakespeare, T. (1994) 'Cultural representation of disabled people: dustbins for disavowal?', *Disability and Society* 9(3): 283–99.

—— (1996) 'Disability, identity, difference', in C. Barnes and G. Mercer (eds) *Exploring the Divide: Illness and Disability,* Leeds: The Disability Press.

—— (1997) 'Defending the social model', in L. Barton and M. Oliver (eds) *Disability Studies, Past, Present and Future*, Leeds: The Disability Press.

Shakespeare, T. and Watson, N. (1997) 'Defending the social model', in L. Barton and M. Oliver (eds) *Disability Studies: Past, Present and Future*, Leeds: The Disability Press.

Silvers, A. (1995) 'Reconciling equality to difference: caring (f)or justice for people with disabilities', *Hypatia: A Journal of Feminist Philosophy* 10(1): 30–55.

Weedon, C. (1987) *Feminist Practice and Poststructuralist Theory*, Oxford: Blackwell.

Wendell, S. (1996) *The Rejected Body: Feminist Philosophical Reflections on Disability*, London: Routledge.

Widdicombe, S. (1993) 'Autobiography and change: rhetoric and authenticity of "gothic style"', in E. Burman and I. Parker (eds) *Discourse Analytic Research: Repertoires and Readings of Texts in Action*, London: Routledge.

Williams, F. (1996) 'Postmodernism, feminism and the question of difference', in N. Parton (ed.) *Social Theory, Social Change and Social Work*, London: Routledge.

Williams, G. (1996) 'Representing disability: some questions of phenomenology and politics', in C. Barnes and G. Mercer (eds) *Exploring the Divide: Illness and Disability*, Leeds: The Disability Press.

Chapter 5

A postmodern perspective on professional ethics

*Amy Rossiter, Isaac Prilleltensky and
Richard Walsh-Bowers*

Introduction

Over the past few years, we have been engaged in research
concerning human service practitioners' lived experience of
professional ethics. The project was stimulated by our concern
about the marginal place ethics occupies in daily professional
practice (Prilleltensky *et al.*, 1996). The outcome of the research has
caused us to think about the nature of the discursive construction of
the field of professional ethics. Our analysis has been informed by
the possibilities that postmodern feminism makes available to social
criticism.

Postmodernism's invaluable and deeply problematic contribution to the human sciences can be summarised through its
declaration of the 'end of innocence' (Flax, 1992). To our minds,
this declaration has opened space for important critical thought in
professional fields like social work or psychology. These disciplines
have traditionally relied on a belief in objectivity as a legitimating
characteristic of the 'special knowledge' that forms the distinction
between professionals and lay people. Postmodernism's insistence
on the connection between power and knowledge ends the
possibility that there can be knowledge that exists independently of
human interests. Such a claim has propelled critiques of the
professions as effects of power rather than bearers of innocent
knowledge deployed to 'help'. These critiques have challenged the
guarantee of progress of professional knowledge by ever-better
scientific foundations, and have instead, raised questions about how
the invention of the human services has taken place (Margolin,
1997; Rose, 1996). The shift from 'real' to 'invention' initiates a

crisis in what we understand counts as professional knowledge, and at the same time, we argue, opens space for aligning professions with a radical democratic project.

The concern to realise the political potential of the postmodern turn has taken us to the work of postmodern feminism. This body of work opposes the charge levelled at postmodernism of inevitable relativism – the idea that denying universal foundations means there is no basis for making ethical judgements. Instead, the thrust of postmodern feminism has been to formulate 'politically engaged critique' (Butler, 1992: 7) that is made possible by postmodernism's understanding of how the 'neutral' foundations developed in modernity (foundations which guarantee professional legitimacy) can be forms of domination which disguise the interests and the power that work through such foundations, as well as through any attempt to oppose those foundations:

> I don't know about the term 'postmodern', but if there is a point, and a fine point, to what I perhaps better understand as poststructuralism, it is that power pervades the very conceptual apparatus that seeks to negotiate its terms, including the subject position of the critic: and further, that this implication of the terms of criticism in the field of power is *not* the advent of a nihilistic relativism incapable of furnishing norms, but, rather the very precondition of a politically engaged critique.
>
> (Butler 1992: 6)

It is feminism's insistence on formulating a political project from postmodern critiques that makes it an important resource for the professions. Feminism's goal is analysis which has the potential to alter our current gender arrangements (Flax, 1990). Human services must also aim towards an analysis of how power works in professions as part of the formulation of practices of freedom, notwithstanding the inevitability of their construction in power. Feminism has taken up postmodernism in order to disturb the roots of patriarchy in modernism – roots which are the legacy of professional knowledge as well. Nancy Fraser and Linda Nicholson ask, 'How can we combine a postmodernist incredulity toward metanarrative with the social-critical power of feminism?' (1990: 34). This is a useful question for those of us who seek to trouble the relation between human service professions and domination. How can we question the foundations of professional knowledge in ways that practise social criticism?

This chapter is an effort to disturb the innocent space professional ethics has traditionally occupied. The goal of such a disturbance is a greater understanding of the way power works in professions as a precondition for the discernment of professional practices that are consistent with social justice. We believe that there is a relation between professional ethics and power that has not been heretofore examined. The consequence of this gap has been the relegation of professional ethics to a marginal place in daily practice. Our task is clarified by Nicholson when she says, 'The task then for contemporary social theory committed to strong forms of democracy is to bring into question any discursive move which attempts to place itself beyond question' (1995: 5).

We believe that our work challenges the conception of professional ethics that has been made by its history within modernism. That conception has been characterised by the assumption that the field of ethics exists in a kind of rarefied space beyond the reach of power, and stands unaffected by its relations to the messy world of practice. Instead, we envision professional ethics as an explicitly political, reflexive effort to understand its own implication within power, and within governmentality. 'It is this movement of interrogating that ruse of authority that seeks to close itself off from contest that is, in my view, at the heart of any radical political project' (Butler, 1992: 8).

Beginning with questions about the centrality of ethics in human services, we wanted to develop ideas about why ethics are lived as encapsulated methods which only come into use during occasions that are formally defined as 'ethical dilemmas'. We assumed that agencies and organisations that are able to enliven ethics in daily practice – to maintain the centrality of ethics – are better able to promote client welfare than agencies where ethics maintains a marginal place. Consequently, we conducted an interview study with personnel from three human service agencies in order to develop descriptions of ethics from workers' lived experiences.

Our discussions with participants caused us to radically question professional ethics as a discursive field. We have come to understand professional ethics as an effect of power which also produces power. Discourses of professional ethics depend on the construction of practitioners as isolated, autonomous individuals – the ideal of liberal humanism – and consequently construct ethics as properly emerging from an internal, private, cognitive function of that individual. In contrast, a postmodern view that suggests that subjectivity is constructed as an effect of power radically displaces the concept of the monadically deliberating subject. Indeed, such a view implies that ethics takes place within a social space that provides the limits and possibilities for individual decision-making. This social space is constructed within the local organisation, in relation to external organisations, within the context of larger social forces, and with reference to the history of human service professions. In other words, ethics are socially constructed within relations of power that influence the centrality of ethics.

In order to illuminate this claim, this chapter will address three areas:

1   the construction of the domain of ethics with respect to its basis in liberal humanism;
2   the interpretation of our research findings in terms of the social relations of ethics;
3   work in progress toward a postmodern conception of ethics.

Liberal humanism and professional ethics

Professional codes of ethics delineate the normative expectations of professions. The professional ethics literature tends to argue for particular methods of operationalising those norms. Our argument makes the claim that codes of ethics and the professional ethics literature do more than the explicit work of rendering values and priorities – they simultaneously create the field of professional ethics itself, while obscuring the process of production. In other words, codes and the ethics literature are discourses that delimit the boundaries around what is properly ethics and what is not. This created object, 'ethics', as the only version available, becomes our taken-for-granted understanding of the sphere of ethics.

In the case of professional ethics in the human services, the discourses of codes of ethics and models of application clearly construct ethics on the basis of liberal humanism. By liberal humanism, we mean the assumption of a unique essence in human beings that is neither contingent nor historical. Liberal humanism understands knowledge as a product of men's ideas, and consequently that social organisation emerges from human nature:

It has imposed a set of assumptions about 'human nature' and 'human freedom' which take it that Man, generally and individually, is the source of knowledge, meaning, history. History, then, is said to result from the action of a *subject*, who is Man, and, as Althusser points out, the thesis is put forward that 'It is man who makes history'.

(Macdonell, 1986: 37)

Professional ethics is founded on the notion that ethics is guaranteed through the rational consciousness of free-willed individuals who may make ethical decisions without reference to history or contingency. For example, the *Canadian Code of Ethics for Psychologists* constructs this notion of ethics in its preamble: 'Responsibility for ethical action by psychologists depends fore-most on the integrity of each individual psychologist; that is, on each psychologist's commitment to behave as ethically as possibly in every situation' (Canadian Psychological Association, 1991: 19). The site of ethics is the individual practitioner who is charged with the necessity of behaving ethically. We read this notion as our natural and normal understanding of ethics.

Similarly, the *Canadian Association of Social Workers Code of Ethics* (Canadian Association of Social Workers, 1994) sets out all of its seventy-seven ethical duties and obligations in entirely individual terms, using the words 'social worker' as the subject of every statement. For example: 'A social worker shall maintain the best interest of the client as the primary professional obligation'. Clearly, at the centre of ethics is the individual social worker, who is the origin of professional ethics.

We are not arguing about the merit of framing codes of ethics in terms of individuals – there may be good reasons, such as accountability, why this is so. However, we are trying to demonstrate that there is a process of production of the field of ethics itself that is actioned through these codes. Understanding that the field of ethics is produced rather than 'natural' allows new insights into its vulnerabilities and greater possibilities for conscious reshaping of the terrain.

The individualism of the codes of ethics is carried further in the professional ethics literature. This literature tends to focus on how to improve, hone, or regulate the subject of ethics – the individual practitioner. Consequently, much of that literature provides prescriptions that are designed to help practitioners make better ethical decisions. With the subject of ethics clearly centred on the individual, prescriptions specify cognitive 'frameworks', which are designed to provide a linear, internal process which, if followed, guarantees an ethical decision. For example, the Companion Manual to the *Canadian Code of Ethics for Psychologists* (Canadian Psychological Association, 1991) details a seven-step plan for resolving ethical dilemmas. It provides examples of dilemmas that are matched to charts which describe the relevant principles and their weight within the code.

Many frameworks provide formulas which match philosophical ethics with practical applications. For example, Woody (1990) provides a model of ethical decision-making which combines ethics theories with professional considerations such as codes, socio-legal concerns, professional theories and professional or personal identity issues. The model is intended to guide individual's reflection process when faced with an ethical dilemma.

The explicit claim of such frameworks is that ethical decisions can be made by individual practitioners when correct cognitive processes are followed. Indeed, Loewenberg and Dolgoff, in a text on social work ethics assert that 'professional social work ethics are intended to help social workers recognize the morally correct way of practice and to learn how to decide and act correctly with regard to ethical aspects of any given professional situation' (Loewenberg and Dolgoff, 1992: 5). Again, we wish to draw attention away from questions of the worth of such frameworks and emphasise instead how our common-sense understanding of what constitutes ethics is produced through discourses of individualism.

In general, that common-sense understanding is that professional ethics consists of an individual practitioner who is the locus of control for ethical decision-making and that the individual's potential to make good decisions can be improved by the provision of cognitive frameworks that can be applied by the individual in occasions of ethical conflicts.

There are a number of studies that attempt to deal with the social context of ethics by looking at individuals within the context of organisations (Cossom, 1992; Kolenda, 1988; Kugelman, 1992; O'Neill and Hern, 1991; Reiser *et al.*, 1987, Smircich, 1983; Trevino, 1986). However, these approaches do not trouble the problem of liberal humanism as the basis for ethics. We therefore want to demarcate some fundamental differences between our approach (Walsh-Bowers *et al.*, 1996) and the orientation of the literature on ethics and organisation.

A good example can be found in Linda Trevino's work on ethics. In her article entitled 'Ethical decision making in organizations: a person–situation interactionist model', Trevino claims that previous approaches to ethical decision making studied either the individual role or situational variables but that 'neither approach has captured the important interfaces among individual and situational variables' (1986: 601–2). She therefore proposes 'an interactionist model that recognizes the role of both individual and situational variables' (ibid.: 602).

In essence, Trevino's proposal draws on Kohlberg's model of cognitive moral development. She posits a relationship between people's moral developmental level, specific individual variables and organisational variables. The individual variables which influence moral decision-making in organisations are ego strength, field dependence and locus of control. The organisational variables are the organisation's normative structure, referent others, obedience to authority, responsibility for consequences, reinforcement contingencies and other pressures.

Trevino's proposal retains the liberal humanist individual as the conceptual base. This individual has particular internal characteristics (stage of development, for example) which determine his or her 'susceptibility' to organisational variables. In fact, Trevino's account posits an 'ideal type' for ethical individuals – one who is least susceptible to 'external' influences. This individual has achieved a post-conventional stage of moral development and has a high level of ego strength, exhibits field independence, and has a strong internal locus of control.

In our view, this ideal type adds up to the autonomous, independent, masculine ideal of the Enlightenment, and it is he who is most removed and unmoved by 'situational variables' and who is therefore most capable of ethical decision-making. With an intact, pre-formed individual who withstands particular effects of organisations, Trevino is unable to deal with the contingent nature of ethics as individuals who are formed in larger social relations continuously construct the ethics of organisations that in turn construct them as moral actors.

It is interesting to note Trevino's failure to consider the issue of power in her formulation. Trevino's construction of the ideal individual who is least susceptible to organisational influences in reality speaks to vulnerability and safety in relation to authority. Trevino assumes that locus of control, field independence, and ego strength are encapsulated individual characteristics that come with the pre-formed individual. In contrast, we advance a position that assumes that such 'characteristics' are products of social relations that are always under construction and that reflect relations of power in organisations and in larger society. Trevino's individual characteristics (post-conventional ethics, field independence, locus of control and ego strength) are psychological descriptors of male privilege. We can assume that white male privilege grounds less vulnerability in organisations, consequently making the exposure of individuality in decision-making more possible. Therefore, our re-interpretation of Trevino's model suggests that gender, race, and class are extremely important variables is producing the safety in organisations, and such safety affects the possibility of voice.

This is not to suggest, however, that privilege sponsors better ethical decision-making. It may, perhaps, produce a sense of being 'one of them' in ways that make conflict or disagreement within a limited frame more possible. However, this very sense of 'being at home' in the authority relations of hierarchies may make a critical vantage point on the ethics of 'home' itself out of reach.

The liberal humanist assumption forms the basis of conventional attempts to understand the relations between individuals, organisations, and ethics. These understandings are predicated on a conceptual division between the individual and the social (Henriques et al., 1984). The individual encounters the organisation with particular characteristics that act on the organisation in particular ways. Thus Kolenda, in his volume on organisations and ethical individualism, speaks about the authors' intent to 'explore various avenues toward a restoration of ethical health in organisations by revitalizing the moral resources of individuals' (1988: xii). Within this conception, problems with ethics neatly dovetail with codes of ethics and the ethics literature – the improvement of the individual is the goal of professional ethics. There are powerful effects of such an understanding of ethics, and those effects are directly related to the limited and boundaried place for ethics in the human services. Chris Weedon, in discussing the general effects of individualism says that 'The liberal-humanist assumption that the individual subject is the source of self-knowledge and knowledge of the world can easily serve as a guarantee and justification of existing social relations' (1987: 84). Weedon is pointing to the notion that we cannot apprehend, and therefore act on, the social relations that produce our experiences when those experiences are viewed as beginning and ending in the individual. In the case of ethics, deploying the individual practitioner as the unit of analysis and action prevents us from acknowledging and analysing the social relations of ethics.

In contrast, our research advances a postmodern perspective on professional ethics which begins from the premise that individuals and organisations are always engaged in a process of construction. 'There is ... no lone individual, no single point of causality, but subjects created in multiple causality, shifting, at relay points of dynamic intersection' (Walkerdine, 1985: 238). This view suggests that the site of ethics is not the independent, pre-formed individual who may be more or less precariously influenced by organisations. The site of ethics, instead, is the process of production of ethical possibilities and limitations within the social relations of the particular location of the ethical concern. Thus, individuals are not 'susceptible' to organisations – they are constantly engaged, within mutually constituting relations with their organisations, in the business of making and being made as ethicists. We wish, therefore, to shift our attention from the internal reflections of individual workers to the social relations which make versions of ethics. It is to a more concrete discussion of these social relations that we will now turn.

Shifting the domain of ethics to social relations

The social relations of ethics

We would like to begin by summarising our findings from research in three human service settings (Prilleltensky et al., 1996; Rossiter et al., 1996; Walsh-Bowers et al., 1996). We will then discuss the implication of our findings for a postmodern conception of ethics. Our qualitative study was based on in-depth interviews with participants in three sites: a general family counselling agency, a hospital department of social work, and a child guidance clinic. In general, when asked to describe their lived experience of ethics, participants talked about the social relations in which their experience of ethics was conditioned. Most participants treated ethics codes as irrelevant and they tended not to employ internal cognitive schemes to resolve ethical dilemmas. Participants saw such resources as esoteric and not useful in the real world of practice. Many participants treated ethics as a compartmentalised professional superego – an overall set of 'shoulds' which, by definition, must be connected to the world of practice. This sense of needing to connect ethics to practice is interesting in that it indicates the degree to which practice and ethics are always/already set apart in language and thought. Indeed, this compartmentalisation is deeply implicated in the marginal place of ethics in human service agencies. It acts as a way of limiting what can be perceived as 'ethics'.

Throughout the course of the interviews, participants talked about their ways of negotiating their practice experiences within systems that conditioned both what they apprehended as 'ethics' and how they responded to ethical conflicts and pressures. In each of the three settings, it was possible to discern a rough picture of the possibilities and tensions which actively worked to condition ethical processes. These pictures are by no means a 'whole story' – they are interpretations that help us to open up the story of ethics to possibilities which might promote a more central place for ethics.

In the family counselling agency, we were told by workers that their ideal method for resolving ethical dilemmas was through dialogue. When confronted with an ethical conflict, they sought trusted colleagues or supervisors in order to engage in conversation which could help them with the subtle work of examining multiple points of view, weighing options, foreseeing outcomes, anticipating reactions and deciding on strategies. However, this kind of conversation requires that participants also deeply examine their own motives, feelings, countertransferential reactions, and political values. This latter requirement of ethics dialogue imposed the need for what workers called 'a safe space'. This space involved an interpersonal context in which workers felt free to make themselves vulnerable in order to deeply examine their own participation within the ethical dilemma.

This 'safe space' was compromised by the organisational dynamics of the agency. As is usual with social work agencies, men were disproportionately represented in management. The agency had suffered extremely serious budget cutbacks, and workers were menaced by job insecurity. Management, particularly during times of financial hardship, tended to use a 'top down' management style that left workers feeling that their professional points of view were ignored in agency decisions. Finally, the hierarchical and paternalistic nature of organisation's management meant that workers would have to expose vulnerability to supervisors who had considerable power over workers' future in the agency. These social relations make the achievement of a 'safe space' for ethical deliberation at best an *ad hoc* interruption of the business of the agency. Workers did not directly link these social relations to ethics, but named them as 'agency politics'. As such, they assumed far less responsibility for politics than they would for the resolution of ethical dilemmas.

In the social work department of a general hospital, we found a different picture of the social relations of ethics. Much the same as the family counselling setting, workers described their need for dialogue about ethics in which they felt that their honesty would not expose them to organisational consequences. The safety of dialogue was jeopardised, however, by the power relations of social work within a medical setting. Our participants told us about interpersonal conflicts with the Director of Social Work and her immediate supervisor. These conflicts tended to curtail interpersonal safety in the setting.

Upon examination, the structure which gave rise to these conflicts involved interacting effects of gender and status in the hospital setting. An all-women social work department within the male-dominated medical system rendered the department vulnerable, particularly in view of the imminent threat of restructuring and downsizing. The Director of Social Work handled this structural vulnerability by trying to monitor workers' conduct so that they did not cause social work's credibility to be questioned. Discourses of professionalism abounded in quite rigid ways. Workers resented this control and attributed it to the personality of the Director, who became the central figure in departmental splits. The personal animosity that thrived in this atmosphere made a 'safe space' for ethics impossible. When workers attributed their fear to the personality of the Director, their own capacity to act as organisational change agents was disabled.

In our third setting, we examined the lived experience of ethics in a child guidance clinic. We talked to psychologists, social workers, and reading clinicians. Because the function of the clinic is to act as a resource to the school system, the social relations of ethics in this case involved relations between the clinic and schools.

Workers identified a shift in the place of professional consultation in the school. Before cuts to the provincial education budget, professionals used to provide assessments primarily viewed within the frame of 'helping children'. With financial threat, the school system shifted the professional's job towards rubber stamping decisions to get rid of troublesome kids. While technical solutions to difficult kids has long been an attractive solution to schools, financial threats limited professionals' ability to challenge such practices. These structural issues were played out at team meetings where relations between teachers, principals, and mental health clinicians became a competition for control of students rather than a process of problem solving. In this dynamic, many ethical dilemmas emerged which, because they involved an external system, were defined as 'politics' which was quite distinct from ethics. Again, 'politics' was treated as something that 'just is' while ethics was seen as requiring professional responsibility.

The three pictures of the social relations of ethics in the settings we studied show both unique and overlapping features. Within each setting, we could discern organisational 'tension sites' which participants identified as they talked about their experience of ethics. These tension sites had their long-range origins in larger social forces – namely the effects of the neo-conservative agenda in Canada, which has called for downsizing and restructuring in health, education, and welfare. These financial pressures acted on organisational forms in which bureaucracy, paternalism, status hierarchies, gender, and external threats interacted with individual investments to produce the social relations of ethics and ethical resolutions. The organisational tension sites were unfailingly marked by fear and threat. They were sites in which dialogue was constrained. In the next section, we will look at how constrained dialogue limits the centrality of ethics in practice.

Power and ethics

In this section, we need to return to Weedon's view that the individualism that extends from liberal humanism tends to obscure the social relations that produce experience. In our view, discourses of ethics that locate ethics in an individual actor who applies cognitive solutions fail utterly to capture the lived experience of ethics described by our participants. In each setting, there are multiple interacting forces that create ethical subjectivities of participants. These subjectivities, forged as they are within power relations, condition what is perceived as ethics, and how ethical dilemmas can be resolved. Yet within the conventional frame of individualism, these complex dynamics which produce the centrality of ethics are perceived as 'politics' – a realm that is set below and outside the purer sphere of uncontaminated individual processes. Thus, the very forces which constrain ethics are kept out of view, and outside the possibility of strategy and action. The inimical result of the separation of power from ethics is blindness to the effects of power on dialogue. It is to these effects that we will now turn.

In his work on ethics, Jürgen Habermas makes a separation between what he calls discourses of justification and discourses of application (1993: 36). Here, Habermas describes a two-step ethical process. The first step, justification, describes a process of determining just norms that is based on democracy and intersubjective recognition. The second step involves the application of those democratically derived norms. Habermas maintains that application of norms must be determined by 'appropriateness' (ibid.: 37) in which the relevant features of practical, local situations are assessed in light of norms. This determination of appropriateness requires complex interpretive deliberation. In other words, application is an interpretive process.

With reference to professional ethics, we can see that professional codes of ethics are the justified norms of the profession. However, the application of those norms is interpretive, and depends on the local and particular features of each situation. Participants in our study were clear that the interpretive aspect of application is best carried out in a dialogical process. Because one's own values, feelings, and attitudes are involved in the application of ethics, the process of dialogue is important in the creation of the interpretation. A partner in dialogue helps us recognise our unconscious investments, our blind spots, unrecognised feelings, or unchallenged attitudes. Because of the importance of dialogue in furthering interpretively derived applications of professional norms, one of the major claims issuing from this study is that the centrality of ethics in human services depends upon the possibility of unconstrained dialogue.

It is here that the problem of power becomes salient. The possibility of dialogue, as a condition of the centrality of ethics, is itself dependent on the existence of relative intersubjective safety.

To allow oneself to be open to challenge, to expose feelings and vulnerabilities requires trusting interpersonal relations.

The organisational tension sites we described in the three settings were sites where interpersonal fear and distrust were generated. These social relations had the effect of diminishing the capacity for dialogue due to fears generated by power differentials. For example, in the family counselling setting, making oneself vulnerable within a hierarchical and paternalistic organisational structure during a time of cutbacks meant that an interpersonal climate of distrust curtailed the centrality of ethics because fear impinged on dialogue. In the hospital setting, when the Director of Social Work attempted to protect the status of social work in a medical setting, her regulation of workers produced interpersonal fear which diminished dialogue. At the child guidance clinic, relations of power between professionals and the school system called up fear and the mobilisation of power as a result of the experience of fear.

When we remove the blinders that arise from the construction of ethics as an individual cognitive act, we are more able to see ethics as part of social relations that condition both the perception of ethics and the interpretive processes that accompany application of ethics. In each of our three settings, ethics was understood as a task that required some knowledge of professional norms and individual deliberation about proper application. With no conception of ethics as social relations, workers labelled the organisational tension sites as 'politics', 'abuse of power', or 'turf wars'. These designations were not accompanied by the same sense of personal responsibility as workers felt they had in relation to ethics. The very conditions for ethics were not perceived as part of ethics and therefore part of one's professional responsibility. Thus, ethics, recognised by professionals as a primary professional obligation, remained partitioned off in a rarefied space of codes and unused cognitive frames, while 'politics' – the social relations of ethics – was experienced as a kind of inevitable, omnipresent irritation that must be accepted as 'part of life' rather than as a professional obligation. We believe that this process contributes to the marginalisation of ethics in human service organisations.

The divorce between politics and ethics was the ground for the marginalisation of ethics in all three research sites. In the family counselling site, workers had not developed strategies for dealing with top-down management other than complaining to peers.

Management talked amongst themselves about workers' 'chronic complaining', yet appeared to have no problem-solving commitments in relation to the issues. In the hospital setting, there were few attempts to address the structural roots of the personal conflicts in the department. Again, we found no pro-active strategies on the part of management to address the demoralisation and distrust that were rampant in the department. In the child guidance setting, political relations between the clinic and the school were cast as inevitable and outside the scope of 'what professionals do'. In all three cases, the tensions that proscribed the unconstrained dialogue necessary to determining application of ethical norms were endured with helplessness and varying levels of frustration.

Towards a postmodern conception of ethics

In the previous sections, we have undertaken to describe conventional professional ethics as a discursive field which depends on the liberal humanist subject. We believe that such discursive practices are unable to account for their relation to power, and to the powerful effects that they induce. Because we understand ethics as a process of production within relations of power, we want to advocate resituating ethics within a radical democratic project. Here, we are using a postmodern analysis to support a political project, as is the goal of postmodern feminism.

At the heart of a postmodern conception of ethics is a shift in our common-sense understanding of ethics as the property of individuals who monadically reflect on dilemmas, to a notion of ethics as the social relations that produce individuals and organisations in ways that limit or potentiate ethical decision-making. This shift has two implications for practice. First, it requires attention to issues of communicative process, and second, it requires a much broader set of activities than is associated with conventional professional ethics.

Based on our data, we argue that when ethics is located in social relations, unconstrained dialogue is a condition for increasing the centrality of ethics. Decisions about the appropriateness of the application of professional norms is best accomplished in a dialogue characterised by openness, trust and mutuality. In our data, workers yearned for this 'safe space' but the particular tension sites of the organisations acted against its achievement. In our view, therefore, ethics is best protected when professionals perceive as their professional duty the responsibility to create relations of inter-subjective respect. This responsibility presents us with nothing less than a radical democratic vision. It requires the examination of organisational forms, including but not limited to bureaucratic and paternalistic structures which may support the misuse of power and authority thus constraining dialogue. It requires us to be chronically suspicious of the operation of power and privilege in our relationships. This is particularly true when relationships include differences based on historical exclusion and marginalisation of groups of people. It requires us to monitor the effect of global political changes on organisations and the individuals who are dealing at ground level with such changes. In short, creating relations of intersubjective respect as a condition for the centrality of ethics requires that we constantly raise the question 'who is frightened to speak and why?' and that we take as our obligation the responsibility to name the fear and its source. In this way, a postmodern account of ethics draws attention to the inherent connection between ethics and freedom.

The child guidance clinic in our study helps us ground this sweeping claim in a practical example. Workers drew our attention many times to the problem of control that arose when sharing responsibility for a child with the school. They described the negative repercussions of this problem on ethical norms of confidentiality and self-determination. Workers' version of ethics was to attempt to make the best decision they could, but they were unable to notice and act on the social relations of these dilemmas. The social relations began with funding cuts to the school system that have their origin in Canada's divestment of responsibility for health, education and, welfare in order to make itself attractive to business. These cuts altered professionals' roles in schools as the school system attempted to rationalise and downsize. The change in roles produced a sense of insecurity for professionals which reduced their capacity to engage in honest dialogue which could lead to strategies which had more ethical outcomes for their clients. It is here where the question 'who is afraid to speak and why' should be the primary question in attempting a process of keeping ethics at the centre of professional practice.

Acting on this question requires a range of activities that must fall under the purview of ethics. It means that strategies to reduce fear in organisations are ethical responsibilities. Confrontation, problem-solving, political engagement and risk-taking are all activities that are necessary to increase the centrality of ethics through promoting unconstrained dialogue. It also means that the responsibility for ethics is spread throughout the organisation and beyond. Managers, for example, must hold themselves accountable for the quality of dialogue in organisations as their responsibility for professional ethics.

The connection between freedom and ethics is enabled by communication. Clearly, a shift to a postmodern account of ethics will require us to attend less to regulating methods of individual reflection and more to intersubjective communication. This may seem a daunting task given the current realities of practice. However, we have models, such as Habermas's communicative ethics (Habermas, 1993) and Simone Chambers' thoughts on requirements for democratic communication (Chambers, 1995). These models are based on the relationship between democratic communication and justice.

There is considerable tension between Habermas's communicative ethics and postmodern feminism. Habermas insists on universalist principle of language which is anathema to postmodernism's anti-foundationalism. Feminists such as Nancy Fraser (1995) criticise Habermas's failure to include gender as a central component of his analysis of public and private spheres. Habermas, on the other hand, describes the project of postmodernism as 'conservatism' because of its failure to account for the libratory potential of modernist projects (1989: xxi). However, postmodernism and Habermas share a rejection of language as a denotive process, arguing instead for language as a discursive performance. Habermas insists that the pluralism that becomes evident when language is understood as constitutive means that forms of democratic will-formation must be developed. He asserts that the process of democratic communication (discourse ethics) best enables the formulation of just norms — norms which cannot be specified in advance of the communicative processes of which they are an outcome. His ideal speech situation sets out the conditions in which just norms can be formulated. These conditions include participation, freedom to speak honestly, and freedom from coercion. In this sense, argues Georgia Warnke (1995), Habermas shares important features of the postmodern feminist project in its demand for the inclusion of difference:

> If we are to recognize the legitimacy of different voices, then we cannot allow any to retain a monopoly on the discussion or to exclude the possibility of listening to others. These standards arise out of a critical pluralism itself, for if we are to learn from interpretations and evaluations other than our own, we must provide the conditions under which they can flourish in the communities to which we belong. This project also requires that as feminists we look for programs, policies, and solutions to our controversies that embody differentiation without cutting off possibilities for change.
>
> (Warnke, 1995: 258)

Seyla Benhabib (1990) emphasises the necessity of a political project in postmodern feminism when she calls the political implications of Lyotard's project 'neo-liberal interest group pluralism' (ibid.). Benhabib sides with Habermas in her rejoinder to Lyotard, arguing that tenets of postmodernism need not lead to 'a vision of politics incapable of justifying its own commitment to justice' (ibid.: 125). Instead, she argues for a comparability between postmodernism and Habermas, saying that postmodernism shifts to 'an epistemology and politics which recognizes the lack of metanarratives and foundational guarantees, but which nonetheless insists on formulating minimal criterion of validity for our discursive and political practices (ibid.).

Simone Chambers provides an example of communicative ethics as a feminist project in her description of the Seneca Peace camp as a 'discursive experiment'. Here, she describes how feminist peace activists adopted strategies of consensual will-formation in order to achieve a radical democratic vision. In our view, such communication is crucial to a postmodern conception of ethics where local, particular, historical, and contingent dilemmas require a constant process of argumentation and interpretation.

We would argue that although democratic communication challenges deeply internalised structures of power, in the end it is an entirely practical activity and one for which workers strive on a day-to-day basis, but without the frame of ethics to validate their efforts as a professional obligation. Given most workers' assessment of monadic reflective schemes, connecting communication, freedom and ethics may well be a more practical method for achieving a central place for ethics in professional practice.

Bibliography

Benhabib, S. (1990) 'Epistemologies of postmodernism: a rejoinder to Jean-François Lyotard', in L. Nicholson (ed.) *Feminism/Postmodernism*, New York: Routledge.

Billingsley, A. (1964) 'Bureaucratic and professional orientation patterns in social casework', *Social Service Review* 38: 400–7.

Butler, J. (1992) 'Contingent foundations: feminism and the question of postmodernism', in J. Butler and J. Scott (eds) *Feminists Theorise the Political*, New York: Routledge.

Canadian Association of Social Workers (1994) *Canadian Association of Social Work Code of Ethics*, Ottawa, Ontario: Author.

Canadian Psychological Association (1991) *Canadian Code of Ethics for Psychologists*, Ottawa, Ontario: Author.

Chambers, S. (1995) 'Feminist discourse/practical discourse', in J. Meehan (ed.), *Feminists Read Habermas: Gendering the Subject of Discourse*, New York: Routledge.

Cossom, J. (1992) 'What do we know about social workers' ethics?' *The Social Worker/Le Travailleur Social* 60(3): 165–71.

Flax, J. (1990) *Thinking Fragments: Psychoanalysis, Feminism, and Postmodernism in the Contemporary West*, Berkeley, CA: University of California Press.

—— (1992) 'The end of innocence', in J. Butler and J. Scott (eds) *Feminists Theorise the Political*, New York: Routledge.

Foucault, M. (1997) *Ethics: Subjectivity and Truth*, ed. P. Rabinow, New York: The New Press.

Fraser, N. (1995) 'What's critical about critical theory?', in J. Meehan (ed.), Feminists Read Habermas: Gendering the Subject of Discourse, New York: Routledge.

Fraser, N. and Nicholson, L. (1990) 'Social criticism without philosophy: an encounter between feminism and postmodernism', in L. Nicholson (ed.) *Feminism/ Postmodernism*, New York: Routledge.

Habermas, J. (1989) *The New Conservatism*, Cambridge, MA: MIT Press.

—— (1993) *Justification and Application: Remarks on Discourse Ethics*, Cambridge, MA: MIT Press.

Henriques, J., Hollway, W., Urwin, C., Venn, C. and Walkerdine, V. (1984) *Changing the Subject: Psychology, Social Regulation and Subjectivity*, London: Methuen.

Kolenda, K. (1988) *Organizations and Ethical Individualism*, New York: Praeger.

Kugelman, W. (1992) 'Social work ethics in the practice arena: a qualitative study', *Social Work in Health Care* 17(4): 59–80.

Loewenberg, F.M. and Dolgoff, R. (1992) *Ethical Decisions for Social Work Practice*, fourth edition, Ithaca, Illinois: F.E. Peacock.

Macdonell, D. (1986) *Theories of Discourse: An Introduction*, Oxford: Basil Blackwell.

Margolin, L. (1997) *Under the Cover of Kindness: The Invention of Social Work*, Charlottesville: University Press of Virginia.

Martin, P. (1989) 'The moral politics of organisations: Reflections of an unlikely feminist', *The Journal of Applied Behavioral Science*, 25(4): 451–570.

Nicholson, L. (1995) 'Introduction', in S. Benhabib, J. Butler, D. Cornell, and N. Fraser (eds) *Feminist Contentions: A Philosophical Exchange*, New York: Routledge.

O'Neill, P. and Hern, R. (1991) 'A systems approach to ethical problems', *Ethics and Behavior* 1(2): 129–43.

Prilleltensky, I., Rossiter, A. and Walsh-Bowers, R. (1996) 'Preventing harm and promoting ethical discourse in the helping professions: conceptual, research, analytical, and action frameworks', *Ethics and Behavior* 6(4): 287–306.

Reiser, S.J., Bursztajn, H.J., Appelbaum, P.S. and Gutheil, T.J. (1987) *Divided Staffs, Divided Selves: A Case Approach to Mental Health Ethics*, New York: Cambridge University Press.

Rhodes, M. L. (1986) *Ethical Dilemmas in Social Work Practice*, Boston: Routledge and Kegan Paul.

Rose, N. (1996) *Inventing Ourselves: Psychology, Power, and Personhood*, Cambridge: Cambridge University Press.

Rossiter, A., Walsh-Bowers, R. and Prilleltensky, I. (1996) 'Learning from broken rules: Individualism, bureaucracy, and ethics', *Ethics and Behavior* 6(4): 307–20.

Smircich, L. (1983) 'Concepts of culture and organisational analysis', *Administrative Science Quarterly* 28: 339–58.

Trevino, L. (1986) 'Ethical decision making in organizations: a person-situation interactionist model', *Academy of Management Review* 11(3): 601–17.

Walkerdine, V. (1985) 'On the regulation of speaking and silence', in C. Steedman, C. Urwin, and V. Walkerdine (eds) *Language, Gender and Childhood*, London: Routledge and Kegan Paul.

Walsh-Bowers, R., Prilleltensky, I. and Rossiter, A. (1996) 'The personal is organisational in the ethics of hospital social workers', *Ethics and Behavior* 6(4): 321–36.

Warnke, G. (1995) 'Discourse ethics and feminist dilemmas of difference', in J. Meehan (ed.) *Feminists Read Habermas: Gendering the Subject of Discourse*, New York: Routledge.

Weedon, C. (1987) *Feminist Practice and Poststructuralist Practice*, Oxford: Basil Blackwell.

Woody, J.D. (1990) 'Resolving ethical concerns in clinical practice: toward a pragmatic model', *Journal of Marital and Family Therapy* 16(2): 133–50.

Chapter 6

Deconstructing and reconstructing professional expertise

Jan Fook

Introduction

It is commonly agreed that the professions find themselves in a time of crisis (Rossiter, 1996). The crisis arises partly from the changes in the contexts in which practitioners profess their profession, but also from the ways in which the professions have responded, or failed to respond to these changes.

As noted in the Introduction to this book, postmodernism can be viewed in two ways: as a characterisation of the current age in which we live, or as a particular style of theorising about our world. Both of these views are of relevance in understanding the current crisis of the professions. The present historical period is seen as uncertain and changing, with fixed and unified ways of ordering the world under question. There are sociocultural, economic, geopolitical and epistemological aspects of these changes, which in broad terms constitute a major upheaval of known and accepted ways. These upheavals therefore constitute major threats to traditional conceptualisations of professionalism and professional practice.

Additionally, postmodernist theorising poses new ways of understanding, and criticising the social phenomenon of professionalism. Whereas traditional criticisms have previously focused on the role of the professions in maintaining structural inequalities, postmodern thinking broadens the critique to understandings of how professionalism maintains power relations through many levels of discourse.

It can be argued, in broad terms therefore, that postmodern analysis is needed to make sense of what can be characterised as a postmodern world (Leonard, 1997). Therefore, in relation to the phenomenon of professional expertise, our analysis needs to cover both an understanding of the postmodern context of professionalism and how it affects the professions, as well as a deconstruction of the notion of professional expertise itself.

What is the precise nature of these criticisms raised through postmodern analysis, and what are the possibilities for professional expertise in the light of them? My main purpose in this chapter is to outline a postmodern feminist analysis of the idea of professional expertise, and to construct, from this analysis and from empirical research on professional expertise (Fook *et al.*, 1999), an alternative conceptualisation of professional knowledge which may be more relevant to the current context, and may potentially challenge and resist relations and structures of domination.

Challenges

What is it about the postmodern world which challenges our notions of professional practice and expertise? Vast global economic changes have resulted in a direct technocratisation (and therefore the devaluing of) professional knowledge and skills. The increased competition brought about through processes of economic globalisation (Dominelli and Hoogvelt, 1996) has increased the pressure to buy and market skills at their cheapest and most measurable levels. The competency movement is a marked example of this (Gould, 1996: 4). In addition, the 'purchaser/provider' split, the new way of organising services so that services are purchased by a body (usually the government) from a 'provider' (usually a smaller community-based or private organisation), apart from increasing competition, effectively removes the power for policy-making from the hands of professionals with specific expertise. Bureaucratic managers maintain control through competitive and short-term contractual funding arrangements.

It is more likely, therefore, that jobs will be short-term, fragmented, and likely to be cast in technocratic or program-based terms, rather than according to professional conceptualisations. For the well-socialised professional, therefore, this entails not only having to compete across traditional professional boundaries for employment, it also means having to market her or himself in de-professionalised ways, often with an emphasis on behavioural skill or ability, rather than theoretical or value base. The crisis, although emanating from economic changes, thus also involves a crisis of meaning, since it is a value base of commitment to service which partially traditionally defines the professions (Greenwood, 1957).

Additionally, the crisis involves a challenge to professional knowledge and control, two other features which are said to define the professions (Friedson, 1970). It is a well-known argument that one way to understand the professions is as occupational groups whose status and identity are defined by their ability to lay claim to, and control, specialised knowledge bases. In this sense, professions are somewhat determined by social context, since the maintenance of their privileged position is dependent on the degree to which they can negotiate social control of knowledge. Professions are socially legitimated by their knowledge claims (Leonard, 1997: 97). In a postmodern world, however, specialist knowledge is challenged as the exclusive domain of a particular professional group. There are at least two aspects of this challenge: a challenge to the authority to generate the knowledge, and a challenge to the authority to *disseminate* the knowledge.

The first challenge thus involves epistemological and social concerns, since it calls into question the types of knowledge which are regarded as legitimate, the ways in which legitimate knowledge is developed, and whose knowledge is regarded as legitimate. Is generalised theoretical knowledge obtained by researchers through scientific rationalist means that which should be the benchmark of professional knowledge? Postmodern thinkers posit that 'grand narratives', or discourses which present a unified voice, are breaking down. In this sense, the search for generalisable and valid theories, which operate regardless of context, is questioned as a valuable or meaningful exercise (Toulmin, 1990).

The dissemination of knowledge also involves similar concerns: who has legitimate authority to dispense professional knowledge and in what ways? Who controls who should be a legitimate member of the profession, and how is this done? Should the ranks of professionals be so tightly guarded and self-protected?

These challenges arise from a broader postmodern movement to question traditional hierarchical arrangements. In this sense the traditional authority of professional knowledge is questioned, as against the legitimacy of the experience of the service-user. Similarly the privileging of the scientific knowledge of the researcher, as against the lived experience of the practitioner, is also debated. Smart (1992: 100) sees professional expertise as 'the citadel

... which has disqualified the understanding and knowledge of "ordinary' people" '.

Implications for social work

There are several aspects of this analysis which are important for social work. Perhaps most importantly, for a profession which prides itself on an integration between theory and practice, postmodern analysis points up a widening gap between the two. The disparities between knowledge and theory generated by professional researchers, and the 'on-the-ground' knowledge embodied in the daily experience of both practitioners and service users are widening. Or perhaps it is not so much that the disparities are widening, as it is that it is now more acceptable to question the taken-for-granted authority of academic researchers. A major set of questions for social work is what constitutes legitimate social work knowledge, how is it best generated, and by whom?

As a follow on from this, we also need to ask whether generalisable knowledge and theories should be the goal of professional research. Will knowledge which is developed to operate regardless of context be meaningful to service users and practitioners? Does the attempt to generate universal knowledge assist the social work endeavour in a postmodern and changing context?

Third, if specialist knowledge is a feature which defines and maintains a position of status for professionals, how is social work to carve out a crucial place when this process of legitimacy is being questioned? What other forms of legitimacy might exist or be developed?

Fourth, the process of professionalisation, particularly for the women's professions, can also be analysed as a process of masculinisation (Hearn, 1992), given that in the transferral of women's caring work from the private to the public domain, women's work is characterised more like men's in order to gain acceptance. In this sense, professionalism can be seen as a type of patriarchal construction, in which male-dominated cultures are privileged. From a postmodern perspective, this is yet another example of how alternative viewpoints and experiences become mainstreamed into one unified view. The main challenge which thus arises for social work, is one of how processes of professionalisation can incorporate, and privilege, different gendered experiences, given that the road to legitimacy is very much defined in masculinist terms.

Finally, from a postmodern perspective, professional thinking in social work exhibits some dangerous modernist tendencies, such as oppositional thinking (Berlin, 1990), and the assumption of static identities in service users (Sands, 1996). Models for professional practice have been constructed on the basis of dichotomising particular categories, often privileging one part of the binary over the other. The privileging of theory over practice is a prime example which causes difficult tensions for students and practitioners (Hindmarsh, 1992). Similarly, diverse groups are often 'othered': characterised, valued and understood in terms of some mainstream norm, which automatically devalues them in relation to the norm. Another worrisome example of oppositional thinking has been the tendency to characterise the public and the personal, the structural or individual, in oppositional terms. Such thinking can lead to a devaluing of the personal, ironic in a profession which ostensibly seeks to reaffirm such values.

In a similar vein, professional practice models are often dependent on a notion of identity which is fixed and not changing. 'Progressive' models of practice assume an ideal of 'strength' towards which the healthy personality works. Such views, however, do not take into account the changing contexts and historical times which all people experience in the course of a lifetime. In this sense, practice models may be far out of touch with the experiences of service users. In relation, then, to professional thinking, social work faces the challenge that many accepted ways of thinking may in fact be outmoded, if not directly inimical to the experiences of diverse groups of service users and practitioners. How then, can professional knowledge be transformed so that it is more directly meaningful and relevant to diverse groups and in diverse contexts?

Challenges for professional expertise in social work

Given the foregoing analysis, the current challenges in developing notions of professional expertise in social work can be summarised as follows. In modernist conceptions, professional expertise is constituted by knowledge which is developed and owned by professional 'experts' who are socially 'licensed' to practise and disseminate this specialist knowledge. The knowledge which is developed tends to be technical, rational and objective, since the scientistic paradigm dominates. This means that there is an emphasis on producing knowledge, or theory, which can be generalised across contexts, and applied in a deductive way to specific situations. In this way, the role of the researcher /academic/theoretician becomes privileged over that of the practititioner and service user, since it is assumed that only knowledge which is generated and used in this way is valid. In a modernist conception, legitimate professional expertise is thus defined as that which is generalisable (acontextual), developed by scientific method by researchers, and applied by practitioners to service users. The culture and processes which are legitimated in this framework tend to be masculinist – practice models tend to reinforce a unified notion of the ideal, diversity is often othered and devalued, the personal becomes silenced.

The challenge in developing notions of professional expertise in social work is one of reconceptualising expertise along postmodern feminist lines, and in so doing, to conceptualise expertise in ways which are more relevant in a postmodern context. Can social work expertise be characterised in ways which are more representative of practitioner and service user experience, many of whom are women? Can knowledge be developed which attempts not so much to generalise, but to be applicable across diverse contexts and with diverse people? Will professional expertise, characterised in this way, still help to legitimise professional standing in a way which contributes to some greater good?

Researching professional expertise in social work

These were some of the questions which motivated some studies undertaken by myself and colleagues Martin Ryan and Linette Hawkins (Ryan et al., 1995; Fook et al., 1996, 1997). Although no one study could hope to address all the issues raised by the foregoing analysis, we were motivated in particular by a desire to know how professional practice was actually experienced in concrete terms by practitioners. We also wanted to know whether it would be possible to conceptualise professional expertise in different ways, based on the experience of practitioners.

In this section of the chapter, I will describe briefly the main findings of this research and then develop these findings into some broad ways in which professional expertise might be conceptualised in feminist postmodern terms. In doing this I am mindful of the arguments put forward by Harding and Flax, which Barbara Fawcett and Brid Featherstone have discussed in Chapter 1 of this volume. Harding (1990) identifies 'standpoint feminism' as a perspective grounded in the belief that women's experiences and perspectives can provide an advantaged viewpoint. It is this advantaged viewpoint which will somehow lead to the challenging of women's oppression. On the other hand, the question remains as to what extent the knowledge derived from women's experiences can be said to be any purer or more innocent, less contaminated by situation or standpoint than any other. A key issue for feminist postmodernists therefore is whether situated and localised knowledge can be conceptualised in such a way as to have more generic significance. Is there an alternative to generalising and universalising, which incorporates diverse voices, but which provides meaning for many?

This is the question I try to address in this chapter, using the experiences of practitioners derived from the research previously mentioned. While our studies were not exclusively focused on women, the bulk of participants were of course women, since social work is a woman's profession. Our intention was twofold, however. First, we did hope that by studying practice from a women's profession, we could include the voice of women in defining notions of professional expertise. Second, our intention was also to focus on the voice of practitioners more broadly, as a group whose perspective is devalued in much professional research. In this chapter I will be attempting, however, not so much to argue that the conceptualisations we developed represent the perspectives of women or practitioners, and therefore should be privileged over current more scientistic representations: indeed, the experiences of women and practitioners are as influenced by dominant discourses as any others. Rather, I wish to use practitioners' current and concrete experiences to reconceptualise notions of professional expertise which are more meaningful to a range of practitioners from diverse situations. By increasing the number of prisms through which we understand our world, I would hope we can increase our understanding of the complexity of experiences in ways which will allow us to act more relevantly.

The study

The main study which is of significance to this chapter was a study of thirty experienced social workers. This has been described fully elsewhere (Fook *et al.*, 1996 and 1999). For the purposes of this chapter I will briefly summarise the study and its findings. Thirty 'expert' social workers were identified by colleagues. Generally, 'experts' met the criteria of having more than five years post-graduation practice experience and having supervised more than five social work students on placement. Colleagues also used their own judgement about who was considered 'expert'. In interviews, each participant was asked to respond to a practice vignette, and to describe an incident from their practice which they considered significant. The design required concrete descriptions of practice, rather than theoretical justifications, since we hoped to obtain a description of the workers' experience in their own words, as far as possible. Transcripts were analysed thematically.

The practice of 'expert' practitioners was also compared to that of beginning and developing practitioners, derived from another study undertaken by us (Ryan *et al.*, 1995). Thus we could begin to draw a picture of how expertise develops over time.

A major theme was the complexity of practice situations, and the ability of workers to handle complexity. They dealt with a range of diverse situations, involving many players, with competing and conflicting interests, yet were able to prioritise important factors quite readily. For example, many workers handled situations in which there were competing interests among service users themselves, and where the question of 'who is the client?' constantly arose, and where there were many different competing clients, who might also change over time, and also according to the perspective taken.

Of relation to the issue of complexity was also the issue of context. They were acutely aware of the influence of differing contexts, particularly workplace, in determining the parameters of their practice. They were aware that different workplaces might require totally different roles or expectations, in some cases contrary to what they perceived as a professional social work role. In many instances they were aware of making distinct choices, in line with either workplace or professional requirements. Involved in the awareness of context in practice, was a heightened sense of limitations and restrictions – not in a negative sense, but in the sense that they were 'realistic' about the variety of factors which might be outside their control. Experts were generally able, through experience, to be aware of contextual factors which they could or could not control, and were able to fashion strategies accordingly.

Another major theme was the lack of formal theory in demonstrated use. Few workers actually articulated a systematic theoretical framework, as taught in social work textbooks, although their talk about their practice did demonstrate the use of isolated concepts, such as 'power'. It was clear though that workers had developed their own frameworks for making sense of what they did, and had recourse to isolated concepts when these appeared meaningful to them. They had clear rationales for their practice – these rationales simply did not fit textbook conceptualisations. This was in direct contrast to students, who tended to apply textbook theories in deductive fashion.

In some instances, workers clearly constructed a process whereby the 'theory' of how to help the service user was generated mutually. One social worker, being uncertain how to respond, simply sat and listened to a woman pour out her feelings for two hours. By responding intuitively, the two engaged in therapy, and the worker developed her own theory about the use of self in a more 'personal', rather than 'professional' way.

This openness to the service user's experience, and the engaging in a process which enables them to communicate it, is related to the decision of some experienced workers not to use preconceived theory, but rather to try to remain as open to the situation as possible and to 'play it by ear'. It was as if they were willing to risk uncertainty for the sake of constructing the most relevant process and outcome for service users. One worker states, in relation to her sense of social work theory: 'each person is creating their own useful practice in allowing clients to experience their own paradoxes and contradictions' (Fook et al., 1999, Chapter 7).

Despite having clear rationales, a sense of uncertainty pervaded many accounts. In the words of another worker:

> There is certainty yet I am comfortable with uncertainty. I have gone from uncertainty and hesitation about my role to developing confidence in that role but also at the same time, to live with uncertainty, which is OK and good; if you stay uncertain, you'll stay striving towards.
>
> (Fook et al., 1999, Chapter 9)

Part of the uncertainty is an uncertainty of outcome, not being committed to a preconceived idea of a desirable outcome. The following quote from a domestic violence worker with service users of non-English speaking background illustrates this well:

> I now say if a woman comes in, 'Tell me what you would like to happen, how would you like me to help you?'. I take a long time listening to what they want. I don't want to go with a preconceived notion that this woman ends up in a refuge.
>
> (ibid., Chapter 7)

Interestingly experts handled the practice vignette in a variety of ways, focusing on different factors, strategies and outcomes. What was common, however, was a marked ability to readily prioritise factors (often according to their own personal and professional experience) and to engage in a process with the situation. This emphasises the importance of process, a way of engaging with the situation, rather than the idea that expertise is defined by the achievement of a specific type of outcome.

Experienced workers, in this sense, were more immediately engaged and involved with the situation – they tended to see themselves as responsible, able to act effectively in the situation. On the other hand, new students tended to remain more detached, trying to analyse the situation objectively and arrive at a 'correct' solution, rather than seeing their own involvement as crucial to the outcome.

In summary, expertise, as demonstrated by experienced professionals, is characterised by an ability to work in complex situations of competing interests, and to prioritise factors in ways which allow clear action. In so doing they are open to change and uncertainty, able to create the theory and knowledge (often in a mutual way with service users) which is needed to practise relevantly in differing contexts, and to locate themselves squarely in these contexts as responsible actors.

Comparing the findings with modernist notions of expertise

The above findings allow us to begin to conceptualise professional practice from practitioners' current experience. It is interesting, first, to compare this experience with modernist notions of professional expertise. Whereas expertise has been predicated on notions of generalisable theory, applied deductively, we find instead that practitioners tend to create their own theory, to be open to different contexts, and not to have preconceived ideas of fixed or desirable outcomes. Practice is thus more contextual, and theory is generated inductively in relation to context.

Modernist conceptions of expertise also assume a detached researcher, able to make objective and rational decisions from a standpoint outside the situation. By contrast, the practice of expert practitioners is characterised by their willingness to be involved as effective agents in the situation. Far from standing outside a situation, it appears as if effectiveness actually necessitates a sense of personal involvement.

The complex and changing nature of practice situations is another feature of professional practice which modernist models of practice appear inadequate to address. For instance, practice models which assume fixed identities, or oppositional ways of categorising service users and workplaces cannot possibly take into account the complex array of competing interest groups involved in many of the situations in which workers practised.

By contrast, experienced workers were highly aware of competing interests, often amongst service user groups themselves, and needed to recognise different perspectives in operation in the same context. The processes by which experienced practitioners engage with situations and service users also do not appear to fit the more 'scientific' orientation indicated by modernist notions of expertise. Rather than entering situations with superior and fixed notions of desirable outcomes, derived from the legitimacy of professional knowledge, practitioners often engage in a mutual process of discovery with service users, in which, together they create and experience the conditions which assist the person, and at the same time, engage in their own process of self-discovery. In this sense, the traditional professional/service user hierarchy is upset. The professional does not use specialised knowledge or expertise to legitimate a powerful position, but rather to create a situation for mutual benefit.

Reconstructing professional expertise

What does this comparison suggest for how professional expertise might look from a postmodern feminist perspective? Some important differences between modernist notions, and the practice experience of professionals are highlighted. Practitioner experience does appear to indicate that they are grappling with much more change, and uncertainty, than is assumed by a modernist model. Practice is more situated, and theory less generalisable, than allowed for in 'scientific' formulations. Outcomes are less fixed or clear than are suggested by more technocratic perspectives.

In the light of these findings, does it make sense to even talk about, and wish to formulate, notions of professional expertise? Perhaps the notion of professional expertise is so implicitly bound up with modernist notions of the professions and their status, that to continue to believe in its desirability is to participate in a perpetuation of its status.

This dilemma is indicative of the dilemma for many postmodern feminists. How do we challenge the structural and generalised oppressions of modernism, yet at the same time recognise and value a diversity of viewpoints and experiences?

Earlier in this chapter I suggested that taking the standpoint of the practitioner might not be enough to reconceptualise professional expertise in ways relevant to diverse groups. To do so might simply privilege the experience of the practitioner, at the expense of other players. There is a need therefore to reconceptualise expertise, taking into account the concrete experience of the practitioner, but also reformulating it in ways which might be meaningful more broadly.

The challenge thus becomes one of using practitioner experience to devise a schema of professional expertise which transforms (rather than simply opposes) existing formulations. To simply devalue professional expertise, or to deny its existence, or to pose it as oppositional to modernist frameworks, might not address the complexities I have argued are inherent in the issue. The task is therefore to devise a way of talking about expertise which values the skills and knowledge being used, but poses these skills and knowledges in ways which can be engaged with by practitioners, service users, and managers alike. The challenge is to propose a new discourse, derived from practitioner experience, but posed in new terms.

Features of professional expertise in a postmodern context

In this section I will outline the broad features of a new discourse about the features of professional expertise. Some of the ideas presented in this section have been developed more fully, and differently, elsewhere (Fook *et al.*, 1999, Chapter 9). My purpose in this section is primarily to relate these features to aspects of postmodern and feminist thinking.

Contextuality is a major feature of professional expertise. This refers to the ability to work in and with the whole context or situation. This ability requires a knowledge of how differing and competing factors influence a situation. In this sense, the main focus of the professional's attention is the whole context, rather than specific aspects or players within it. The expert simply understands that the pathway to understanding is to understand the whole context, and the differing perspectives which are part and parcel of this. Similarly, the pathway to relevant practice is through working with the whole context. This orientation of contextuality involves a type of connectedness, as discussed by Belenky *et al.* (1986: 113), in which the knower recognises the need to connect with the viewpoints and experiences of others on the road to self-knowledge and learning.

Knowledge and theory creation are related to contextuality in that it involves the ability to generate knowledge and theory which is relevant to changing contexts. This means that experts are constantly engaged with situations so that they are not just modifying existing knowledge, but are in fact creating new knowledge which is relevant to newly experienced, and often changing situations. As Eraut (1994: 54) points out, the skill of using knowledge relevantly in a particular situation involves the skill of creating new knowledge about how to do this. The ability to create new knowledge relevant to context is a skill which can therefore readily be transferred across contexts. The feature of transferability is therefore a major alternative to that of generalisability. What becomes important to the expert practitioner is the extent to which knowledge can be transferred, and made contextually relevant rather than generalisable. In more modernist conceptions, abstract generalised theories are deductively applied to make meaning of newly encountered situations. Existing meanings are imposed. In a more postmodern conception, meaning is created inductively from the experience at hand.

Since the creation of meaning becomes an important skill, this places emphasis on the processual nature of professional expertise. Expert practitioners generally do not foreclose on interpretations or outcomes. Instead, practice and theory are often mutually negotiated with players in the situation.

If knowledge and theory creation are integral features of professional expertise then skills of reflexivity and critical reflexivity are also involved. Reflexivity, in one sense, is related to the skill of theory creation as embodied in the reflective process first discussed by Argyris and Schön (1976). They argued that theory is embedded in practice, and that practitioners therefore develop theory inductively out of ongoing experience. It is this theory which can be articulated and better developed through a reflective process. Professional expertise therefore involves the ability to reflect upon, and develop theory from practice. However, reflexivity refers also to the ability to locate oneself squarely within a situation, to know and take into account the influence of personal interpretation, position and action within a specific context. Expert practitioners are reflexive in that they are self-knowing and responsible actors, rather than detached observers. They are critically reflexive if they also hold a commitment to challenging power relations and arrangements (Fook, 1999). From a postmodern feminist perspective, then, critical reflexivity is a crucial feature of professional expertise.

A tension that practitioners grapple with is how to retain meaning and a broader sense of purpose, when contexts change, and are often contradictory. How does the expert practitioner maintain the will to constantly recreate theory, and keep themselves open to new situations, all the while juggling conflicts? In a broader sense, these are the same questions that postmodernists pose. How do we keep the faith to attain a collective 'good', at the same time not foreclosing on what that good might be by incorporating diverse and conflicting perspectives?

An answer perhaps lies in a pathway that many of our experienced practitioners had forged. Experts appear to subscribe to a broader level of values which transcends the immediate workplace. It may take the form of a commitment to the profession, to social justice ideals, or to a system of humanitarian and social values. Elsewhere this has been termed a 'calling' (Gustafson, 1982), which encapsulates the moral vision of social work. This commitment to a higher order of values allows workers to maintain a grounded yet transcendent vision. It allows them to be fully aware of, and responsive to the daily conflicts of practice situations, yet also allows them to pursue broader goals which make the daily dilemmas meaningful. It might be said that they have developed a construct of professional social work expertise which allows for uncertainty and conflict, and also for a sense of ultimate direction. They are aware of constraints, but like some of the students in Hindmarsh's study (1992: 232), are not disempowered by this awareness. They can act as involved and participating players because they have a meaning system which makes it worthwhile.

In a time of postmodern crisis we need to frame professional expertise as grounded and contextual, involving transferable (rather than generalisable) knowledge and the ability to create this through reflective and reflexive processes. In this way expert professional social workers are able to create critical knowledge which potentially challenges and resists current forms of domination, and they are able to maintain commitment to a system of social values which allows them to work with, yet transcend the contradictions and uncertainties of daily practice.

Bibliography

Argyris, C. and Schön, D. (1976) *Theory in Practice: Increasing Professional Effectiveness*, San Francisco: Jossey-Bass.

Belenky, M., Clinchy, B., Goldberger, N. and Tarule, J. (1986) *Women's Ways of Knowing*, New York: Free Press.

Berlin, S. (1990) 'Dichotomous and complex thinking', *Social Service Review* March: 46–59.

Dominelli, L. and Hoogvelt, A. (1996) 'Globalisation and the technocratization of social work', *Critical Social Policy* 47: 45–62.

Eraut, M. (1994) *Developing Professional Knowledge and Competence*, London: Falmer Press.

Fook, J. (1999) 'Critical reflection in practice and education', in B. Pease and J. Fook (eds) *Transforming Social Work Practice: Postmodern Critical Perspectives*, London: Routledge.

Fook, J., Ryan, M. and Hawkins, L. (1996) 'Expertise in social work practice: an exploratory study', *Canadian Social Work Review* 13 (Winter): 7–22.

—— (1997) 'Towards a theory or social work expertise', *British Journal of Social Work* 27(2): 399–417.

—— (1999) *Professional Expertise: Practice, Theory and Education for Working in Uncertainty*, London: Whiting and Birch.

Friedson, E. (1970) *The Profession of Medicine*, New York: Dodd Mead.

Gould, N. (1996) 'Social work education and the crisis of the professions', in N. Gould and I. Taylor, (eds) *Reflective Learning for Social Work*, Aldershot: Avebury.

Greenwood, E. (1957) 'Attributes of a profession', *Social Work*, 2(3): 44–55.

Gustafson, J.M. (1982) 'Professions as 'callings'', *Social Service Review* 1(56): 501–5.

Harding, S. (1990) 'Feminism, science and the anti-enlightenment critiques', in L. Nicholson (ed) *Feminism/Postmodernism*, New York: Routledge.

Hearn, J. (1992) *Men in the Public Eye*, London: Routledge.

Hindmarsh, J. (1992) *Social Work Oppositions*, Aldershot: Avebury.

Leonard, P. (1997) *Postmodern Welfare*, London: Sage.

Rossiter, A. (1996) 'Finding meaning for social work in transitional times: reflections of change', in N. Gould and I. Taylor (eds) *Reflective Learning for Social Work*, Aldershot: Avebury.

Ryan, M., Fook, J. and Hawkins, L. (1995) 'From beginner to graduate social worker: preliminary findings from an Australian longitudinal study', *British Journal of Social Work* 25(1): 17–35.

Sands, R. (1996) 'The elusiveness of identity in social work practice with women: a postmodern feminist perspective', *Clinical Social Work Journal*, 24(2): 167–86.

Smart, B. (1992) *Modern Conditions, Postmodern Controversies*, London: Routledge.

Toulmin, S. (1990) *Cosmopolis*, New York: Free Press.

Chapter 7

Researching into mothers' violence

Some thoughts on the process

Brid Featherstone

Introduction

In 1993 I began researching into mothers' physical violence towards their children. This chapter was begun some time ago and is part of an ongoing attempt to think through some of the issues that have arisen in the course of this research which primarily appear to concern the relationship and interrelationship of topic, theory and method. It will attempt to interrogate the biographical, theoretical and practical conditions which have enabled and constrained my relationship with the topic and the research method chosen. The 'fit' between theory and method will be a particular concern, reflecting both the importance this has begun to assume in my own work but also a wish to contribute to feminist debates in this area.

This article is therefore an attempt to look at the possibilities, tensions and difficulties within and between my topic, my method and my theoretical perspective. The topic itself raises its own obvious difficulties which were anticipated and, to some extent, planned for and these will be discussed. However, what was not anticipated was the tension between theory and method. The method, that of interviewing women, was chosen at a particular point in time when certain theoretical conditions pertained within debates on feminist research. Its impact on later theoretical developments, in particular the author's shift from a perspective influenced by socialist feminism to one which has allegiances with postmodernism and psychoanalysis (Flax, 1990; Hollway, 1989) has opened up questions which are not just pertinent to this research but also wider debates within feminist research.

In order to ensure some element of coherence in this chapter I will explore the issues in the following order, although it is clear that their interrelationship renders any such order arbitrary and problematic. I will look at the relationship between biography, theory and topic, before moving on to look at that between topic and method and theory and method.

A suitable topic for a feminist?

The relationship between biography, choice of topic and choice of theory is an important one in my view. This is complex territory obliging one to engage with questions of how one reads/construct's one's past and present. I have come to realise in a very 'real' sense that one cannot assume 'any straightforward relationship between theorizing and experience' (Flax, 1993: 3). All narratives are constructed, shaped and constrained by the conventions available.

Exploring my own journey would appear to indicate that under-standings of one's past are indeed provisional and fluid. For example, I have one story about my past – a story which has profoundly affected my choice of topic and the feminist theories I am attracted to. In a world ruled by men I grew up surrounded by strong women who encouraged me to believe that I had every right to belong and achieve. I had little experience of constraint until I entered social settings as an adolescent where I became aware that being pretty was definitely more important than being clever.

My engagement with feminism at university was not experienced as a comfortable homecoming but, rather as a continuation of relationships with women which have been complex, shifting and ambivalent. Growing up I encountered specific women's strength and their anger. In particular I learned about the myriad of ways in which mother/daughter relationships expressed ambivalence whereas, by contrast, relationships with fathers were, in my case, characterised by absence (my father died when I was young). Relationships with other girls, including siblings, were the source of both joy and anguish.

Encountering feminism, at university, did help with the world I was then involved in – a world dominated by what appeared to be clever men and impenetrable ideas – but was less helpful in terms of understanding the world I had grown up in. There were big gaps in feminism for me from the outset. I was aware, for example, of finding little to interest me in feminist approaches which portrayed women as either innocent or powerless or men as straightforwardly powerful.

As a social worker in the 1980s I found the writings of socialist feminists such as Segal (1987) and Gordon (1986 and 1989) seemed to speak both to my understandings of my own life but also to what I was finding in my work. As a social worker, initially with young women who were involved with the criminal justice system, and latterly in the field of child protection, I felt that they and I were positioned in complex and shifting ways in relation to each other, men, children and power.

The issue of mothers' violence towards their children was for me, therefore, a topic in which I could pursue many of the concerns which had preoccupied me for many years. It offered the potential to look at anger, pain, power and powerlessness and it allowed me to explore an issue which had been relatively neglected (Gordon, 1986). It also offered me the opportunity to experience and reflect on a range of feelings; anxiety about the choice of topic being seen as politically incorrect, alongside feelings of defiance in my ongoing and ambivalent relationship with feminism and other women, alongside feelings of concern that sanitised accounts of women leave actual women, particularly those who break the rules, very vulnerable.

What I have described in terms of 'personal biography' has both been reflected in and been replayed in feminist theoretical debates in the 1980s and 1990s. I identified as a socialist feminist for many years. The work of Segal (1987) articulated my own disquiet about the demonisation of men and consequent idealisation of women prevalent in much of feminism in the late 1970s and much of the 1980s. I found her then unfashionable assertion that women exercise power and are not innocent victims very affirming. She reasserted the importance of deconstructing categories such as women and men and working with differences of class and 'race' as well as gender.

Revisiting the above story of 'my life' now after engaging in the research I have done and at this point in time makes me aware of the 'silences' I have engaged in. Why do I not talk about the male teacher who made me feel 'silly' – the women who were clearly struggling – the men who drank all the family budget? I am also left with questions about 'why' the investment in the above story – other women would have used similar circumstances to either engage in radical feminism or alternatively not to find feminism relevant at all.

Like others in the 'postmodern' landscape of the 1990s I find myself interested in moving away from grand narratives, exploring power/knowledge relations and questions of difference. Some writers such as Flax (1990) have named much of what I described earlier and have made it acceptable to be ambivalent, to appreciate subjects as being multiply positioned rather than fixed as good/bad, violent/peaceful. Studying gaps in feminist theory is seen by feminist postmodernists as important rather than embarrassing, a source of interest rather than of censure. In particular, encountering writers who have engaged with feminism, postmodernism and psychoanalysis has led to an appreciation of how repression and displacement can inform all our practices including those of a 'theoretical nature'.

I have been made particularly aware of the dangers of replacing one set of stories about women with another which poses some sort of singular truth. I now recognise, for example, there were points in my research where I was seeking to replace stories of women's powerlessness with stories of their power. In certain interviews I struggled to hear certain kinds of stories because of my anxiety to hear others. There is ample corroboration, for example, in the first few interviews I completed of feminist concerns about male violence. In struggling not to repress those and highlight other areas which have been relatively neglected, I have had in Opie's (1992) phrase to think against myself, to interrogate myself and the process in an ongoing way. Postmodernist suspicions of coherent, integrated and seamless theories have helped in developing this attitude. As McRobbie (1993) notes the value of postmodernism is that it is rude and impertinent in that it shows where power resides, hidden, quiet and displeased at being exposed. Demonstrating these ruses does not mean descending into unruly chaos. Rather, it allows for open debate and dispute about boundaries and discipline and what constitutes a study, what is knowledge (ibid.: 137).

Changing theoretical allegiances have, in my view, enriched the understandings I bring to the research topic. The relationship between topic, theory and the method I adopted is, however, more problematic.

A question of method

When I was choosing my research method, a number of years ago, feminist research writings contained a number of orthodoxies (Maynard, 1994, Kelly *et al.*, 1994). As Maynard notes, the use of qualitative methods which focus more on the subjective experiences and meanings of those being researched was regarded as more appropriate to the kinds of knowledge that feminists wished to make available as well as being more in keeping with the politics of doing research as a feminist. Semi-structured or unstructured interviewing has been the research technique most often associated with this stance although this can produce both quantitative and qualitative data (Maynard, 1994: 12).

Kelly *et al.* (1994), in the same volume, express concern about the growth of an orthodoxy that feminist research or feminist method must involve face-to-face interviewing. They situate their questioning within a project which critically examines what they see as statements which have become key definers of feminist research. These are: feminist research is research on and with women; feminist research uses qualitative methods; it should be empowering for participants and directed towards social change. By contrast, they argue that what makes research feminist is not the methods used but the framework within which they are deployed. There are many occasions, they argue, where research on men is a very valid activity for feminists to engage in. Furthermore, face-to-face interviewing may not be suitable for a range of topics, particularly those where sensitive distressing material is being dealt with.

Not only has it often been assumed that face-to-face interviewing is essential to feminist research, there have also been prescriptions, which have gradually been challenged, about how such interviewing should be carried out. In an influential article Oakley (1981) argued that interviewers should invest their own personal identity in the research relationship and develop reciprocity, intimacy and sometimes long-term friendships. She argued that intimate, non-hierarchical relationships between feminist researchers and those researched could be developed through exploring and invoking their common experiences as women. Oakley's work influenced a generation of feminist researchers.

Cotterill (1992), in her study of mothers-in-law and daughters-in-law, for example, based her methods of interviewing and establishing relationships on the methods advocated by Oakley. She was also influenced by Cornwell's discussion of public and private accounts in interview and the significance of the 'best face' phenomenon. In her attempts to move people from public to private accounts she used multiple interviews designed to develop

> high levels of trust and confidence in the research relationship. Repeated interviewing can also develop the personal relationship between interviewer and interviewee to a point where private dialogue results and frequently leads to what Oakley calls a 'transition to friendship'.
>
> (Cotterill, 1992: 596)

As a result of her experiences in using this approach Cotterill expresses considerable dissent about prescriptions such as Oakley's. She argues that many women find it easier to talk to a researcher precisely because she is a stranger rather than a friend. Furthermore, respondents welcome the opportunity to talk about themselves rather than engage with the researcher's own views or feelings. Cotterill argues for the importance of deconstructing the notion that women respondents will have similar needs and require similar things from the researcher. She also talks about the tensions which arise between the multiple positionings of a researcher as woman, researcher and friend. She alongside others (for example, Stacey, 1991) explores the potential for abuse and exploitation inherent in situations where respondents build up high levels of trust and reveal material which they may regret which is then written up. 'The "sympathetic listener" who seeks to equalize the relationship between herself and her respondents may only succeed in making them more vulnerable' (Cotterill, 1992: 598). In the research literature generally this has been referred to as the problem of informed consent (Lee, 1993). What exactly are people agreeing to when they consent to an interview?

It is now acknowledged that Oakley's approach can be read as an exemplar of a period where differences between women were either not acknowledged or assumed to be amenable to incorporation within a more general commonality around gender position. Furthermore, it is argued that Oakley overestimated the power of the researcher in the research situation and underestimated the issue of power in the wider world.

However, in choosing my own research method I did not seriously consider any other method apart from face-to-face interviewing. In carrying out my first set of pilot interviews I became aware of a number of issues which I wish to contribute to the above debates. They concern two areas: interviewing and its suitability for certain topics and interview practices.

Topic suitability

Mothers' violence towards their children would appear to fit Lee's definition of sensitive research. Such research is 'research which potentially poses a substantial threat to those who are or have been involved in it' (1993: 4). Although he stresses the importance of locating threat contextually, thus avoiding a checklist approach, he does identify threat within three broad areas. The first is where the research poses an intrusive threat in the sense that it deals with areas that are stressful and/or private (for example, bereavement). The second relates to research into communities which are stigmatised or produced as deviant, where there is a possibility that the research might further those processes. Finally, research can be threatening if it impinges on political alignments in the sense of threatening the vested interests of powerful people or institutions (Lee, 1993: 4).

In my view, research into mothers' violence towards their children is threatening in at least the first two areas. It is concerned with areas which are often emotionally stressful. Furthermore, the research can be promoted or used in ways which can have unhelpful consequences for the women concerned and women more generally. Indeed Gordon (1986) has argued that the fear of how it might be used has been a factor in discouraging women from undertaking this research at all, hence the paucity of feminist work in this area.

Depth interviewing has been identified as a suitable method for researching into areas of emotional threat (Brannen, 1988; Lee, 1993). This, alongside the feminist preference for interviewing, has ensured the proliferation of studies into areas such as breast cancer (Cannon, 1989), mother-in-law/daughter-in-law relationships (Cotterill, 1992) and mothers of children who have been sexually abused (Hooper, 1992). Kelly et al. (1994), as I indicated earlier, have questioned this and argue that well-structured questionnaires may be more appropriate, particularly in enabling respondents to disclose difficult material at their own pace.

My own initial experiences of interviewing lead me to suggest that there is a more valuable discussion to be had about the conduct and practice of interviews rather than whether one should or should not interview. In other words the 'how' of interviewing deserves more attention. In my pilot interviews I adopted an unstructured approach and I used certain types of questions which I now recognise as particularly unhelpful both in relation to the demands of the particular topic but also more generally.

The approach was unstructured in the following ways, for example, I constructed an interview guide rather than a schedule (Fielding, 1993). A guide indicates that there are broad areas you want to cover rather than specific questions you want to ask. I did not refer explicitly to the guide throughout the interviews but used the interview to get the woman to talk about what had happened with her child and to reflect on 'why'. In using 'why' I was following a feminist approach. Kelly *et al.* (1994) argues that 'why' is a fundamental and basic feminist question. 'Exploring with individuals why they think and act as they do enriches our understanding, and is a far stronger base from which to explore potential change than knowing only what they think and do' (ibid.: 39).

I would like to address the question of structure and process initially. While it is recognised that developing structures is a defence and can reflect a desire to avoid uncomfortable and painful feelings, it is also recognised that defending against anxiety is an important aspect of our well-being. Some attention has been paid to this issue in relation to the way child protection systems function and there is increased recognition that the endless search for foolproof procedures which has characterised child abuse inquiries in the UK is symptomatic of the painful and distressing emotions that child abuse evokes. There has been less attention paid by feminists to issues of structure and the difficulties plus the safeguards they offer within the research setting. Furthermore, there has been little recognition (particularly within the feminist literature) of the possibility that transference/counter-transference relations might operate within this setting. These particular omissions may have serious consequences.

I found the lack of structure a problem for me in the following ways. It meant that painful material was not contained clearly, there was no clear lead up to it nor was there any winding down from it for either myself or the respondent. I have noted this has meant for other interviewees that interviews can last from four to five hours. As Brannen (1988) has noted, researchers endure conditions that no therapist would.

The effect on me was that I withdrew from the material rather than the actual interview in the sense that I became physically unable to transcribe the tapes. For some of the interviewees there also appeared to be a withdrawal in the sense that they did not attend for second interviews. Sayers (1991) has addressed some of the ways in which counter-transference reactions in male and female social workers can impact on the ways in which cases of abuse are dealt with. Laslet and Rapoport (1975) have looked at transference and counter-transference issues in relation to research. There is as yet little indication that this has been seen as important within feminist research approaches. I personally found that interviewing women about their violent relationships with their children bought up profound feelings of distress and anxiety about my own childhood. I had some of the reactions that have been noted in social workers, for example, hostility and the desire to rescue. I was also aware, in retrospect, that I had to hold and contain interviewees' own feelings of pain and anxiety. It is not just as researchers such as Brannen (1988) and Hooper (1992) recognise that the content of what people tell you is painful but the process itself engages you and them with very deep early memories and anxieties.

Through an increased engagement with feminists who are influenced by postmodernism and psychoanalysis (e.g. Flax, 1990 and Hollway, 1989) I have been able to reflect on and understand the actual process rather than either react or become overwhelmed although I did both those things at times. This has been even more important at the analysis stage which I will deal with later.

My difficulties were further compounded by my use of 'why' questions which in retrospect signalled a number of contradictory things. They signalled an assumption that there was a truth behind women's actions which sympathetic questioning could unveil. Consequently it assumed a rational, unitary subject. Furthermore, as has been generally recognised in social work and counselling circles, the use of 'why' can be experienced as persecutory and is therefore particularly unsuitable for research such as mine where women do already feel in the words of one of my respondents 'like monsters'.

. What may be more helpful, which I am now discovering, are invitations to women to tell their side of the story or simply to tell their story. This can be particularly important where there have been multiple stories constructed within a range of settings such as the court setting and case conferences, and with a range of professionals such as solicitors and social workers. Women very often feel their stories have no space to be heard in many of the settings although I did get a certain sense as Philp (1979) argued that there is a recognition of the ambiguous role social workers can play here. Philp has argued that the role of the social worker historically has been to turn the offender into a subject and to reveal their underlying humanity to the courts. Women did feel able to comment on how well that was done. There was also a clear acknowledgement by one woman of how she had actively worked to produce one version of her story which gave the professionals what she felt they wanted and which would ensure a more favourable outcome for her.

In making the move towards story telling one is signalling a move away from the search for a factual truth or the search to discover what really happened. It fits more closely with my leanings towards postmodernism and helps to deal more easily with contradictions in accounts and behaviour. For example, after interviews I was made aware on a few occasions of other material which cast doubt on the 'veracity' of what I had been told or seemed to completely contradict what I had been told. Initially this caused me great discomfort because I now recognise I was caught in a framework which set up the woman as the privileged source of her truth and wanted to protect her from all those nasty people who disbelieved her. One woman, for example, gave me a very moving account of the loss of her children to the care system and of her great hopes for the baby she was carrying and her determination to give this child and herself a completely fresh start. As a childless woman myself, I found her account poignant and found myself wanting to rescue her and ensure that everything could be done to help her keep this child. When I discovered that she had made other choices later which actively jeopardised this I was initially very thrown. However, in reframing the research act as that of constructing a narrative and moving away from 'why' with its connotations of unitary, rational subjectivity, I am now able to see the interview process as reflecting an aspect of her contradictory positionings.

Analysing data

Reflexivity is crucial at all stages of the research process but is foregrounded at the analysis stage in my view. The many possible ways of interpreting data confront one with important ethical questions as well as questions around 'validity'. Furthermore, if one has a theoretical perspective which is influenced by psychoanalysis then a range of further issues are raised about the status of the account and how one interprets it.

The most common method of analysing qualitative data appears to be coding derived from grounded theory approaches (Strauss and Corbin, 1990) and many feminists appear to use this (Holland and Ramazanoglu, 1994). This involves paying very close attention to the data and generating codes or indexing (Mason, 1996). Initially, I found this useful particularly for earlier interviews. However, particularly when I moved onto a story telling approach it became more problematic. Staying at this level lost a sense of chronology in the sense of allowing an understanding of how mothering is a process which operates across time and space. Also, it does not easily allow for any analysis of what an individual is trying to accomplish through the telling of the story. Furthermore, as Hollway (1989) points out, the cutting and pasting involved can lose the 'integrity' of the case-study as a whole. So although I continued to use coding as a means of getting to grips with the material I did move onto a method very loosely based on that developed by Rosenthal (1990) where I 'tracked' the narrative as a whole exploring how the story unfolded and how continuities and discontinuities emerged and what these appeared to signify.

Here, I want to focus on how shifts in my theoretical position 'enriched', in my view, how I read interview texts. As I have already indicated, the work of Opie (1992) was important in encouraging me to think against myself, interrogate my own positions and seek to ensure that I was not, as far as possible, bending the data to meet my own theoretical or political purposes. Postmodern approaches fostered a useful scepticism towards searching for causes for mothers' behaviour or attempts to find an underlying truth behind the narrative. It also allowed for a range of readings of texts which although potentially overwhelming allowed a 'richer' picture to emerge.

To give an example, I met with one mother who at the point of interview had left her children with her husband and was living separately. She positioned herself variously through the interviews –

as a woman who had lost her sense of 'self' through the process of mothering, as someone who had a strong sense of 'self', and a very precarious sense of 'self'. In relation to her husband she presented as both a 'victim' particularly of his intransigence and potential physical violence and as someone who was in charge particularly in terms of being more emotionally and verbally articulate than him. Her relationship to dominant discourses around motherhood was also complex and contradictory. Her rejection particularly of other mothers and their 'advice' while articulated confidently often betrayed considerable anxiety which resulted in her withdrawing from them.

Psychoanalytic understandings allowed me to recognise that although the narratives she developed were often very 'logical' and coherent, there were points of considerable tension and pain evidenced in changes in tone and physical behaviour. They also alerted me to an appreciation of the variety of emotions both listening to and analysing her story evoked in me.

Opie (1992) argues that sociology has traditionally valorised quantity in terms of data but that data which only occurs momentarily can be crucial in understanding desire and motivation (see White, 1998, however, for a discussion of this). At one point the status of what was not said at all became an issue for me. For example, one woman in an initial interview about her life with her children never mentioned her own childhood at all. I found this significant, but is it? Perhaps she was so engrossed in telling me about the present that the past was not relevant at that point. I, however, have a theoretical position which links how one was mothered with how one mothers. I did, on second interview, go back and discuss this with her but was still aware at the end of that interview that I was interpreting her childhood quite differently to how she described it. Furthermore, when she was exploring her physical violence to her son she started to talk about her anger with her husband even though he had not appeared in the narrative at all until then. The narrative had been almost solely concerned with the difficulties she had experienced in her relationship with her son and with mothering generally. I found it possible to read this in a number of ways. The lack of mention of her husband up until this point could relate to the way she chose to tell the story and build up a picture for me of her oppression. It could also be read as an attempt by her to avoid getting in touch fully with her feelings of anger towards her son by deflecting them onto her husband – a more acceptable position for a feminist which is how she wished to portray herself to me.

The above brief look at analysing data is an attempt to highlight some of the issues which arose for me. Issues around analysis, in common with attention to wider concerns in research, are becoming the subject of considerable attention in feminist research writings and also in social work research writings (see White, 1998). The recognition by researchers of the importance of identifying and questioning ideology – not just the ideology of the researched – but also one's own is a very welcome development in my view. Open discussion about the dilemmas involved in analysing is also welcome.

A word on the fit between theory and method

As I indicated at the onset, the ordering of this chapter is to some extent arbitrary and problematic. Clearly, in the last section I was discussing issues of theory and method as well as topic and method. In this section I want to make some brief points about some of the general issues about the relationship between theory and method. The feminist research literature often does not refer explicitly to theory when identifying the different stages or aspects of the research process. Method, methodology and epistemology are the terms used. Maynard (1994) notes that Harding's distinction between these terms is generally recognised as very helpful.

> [Method] refers to techniques for gathering research material, methodology provides both theory and analysis of the research process. Epistemology is concerned with providing a philo-sophical grounding for deciding what kinds of knowledge are possible and how we can ensure that they are both adequate and legitimate.
>
> (Maynard, 1994: 10)

Theory becomes subsumed within methodology here.

The disappearance of theory as a distinct aspect of the research process has occurred alongside and is more than likely related to the disappearance of the practice of using certain theoretical frame-works to characterise particular types of feminism (e.g. radical feminism, socialist feminism). Furthermore, there has been an increased tendency to use the generic term feminist to describe one's orientation thus obscuring rather than clarifying one's beliefs about a range of issues. Alongside this has developed an assumption that postmodernism is of concern only at the epistemological level and has little to do with concrete research practices.

I now want to argue in this last section that the above developments are not helpful either in developing rigorous research practices or in ensuring that the process is seen as rigorous. It is vital that researchers clarify as far as possible what kinds of theories they hold, how these shift and change and how these affect what they do and how they do it. For example if we retrace the steps I have taken in this chapter it is possible to see that I developed my research and my research method while influenced by certain versions of socialist feminism (e.g. Segal, 1987 and Gordon, 1989) which clearly allowed certain questions to be posed relatively easily. These concerned mothers' ability to be violent and to be powerful. Furthermore, it was easier to explore the differences between women and between men.

However, it arguably closed down questioning in certain areas which had implications for method in particular. Such questions in particular concerned understandings of subjectivity. For socialist feminism was still largely caught up with beliefs that subjectivity is rational and unitary. Developing postmodern and psychoanalytic understandings enabled a move away from this and helped to foster an increased and proper reflexivity about the process. As I indicated earlier it fostered the conditions in which it is possible to 'think against yourself'.

This is particularly important to state in the current context where as I indicated earlier postmodernism is seen as an epistemological issue. This means that writers like Kelly *et al.* (1994) can dismiss it as far removed from 'the practical concerns which preoccupy researchers: how to get access; how to build a sample; what methods to use; what questions to ask and how to word them; how to make sense of the information we have collected. If taken in its strong form postmodernism suggests that most recognised forms of social research are pointless exercises' (Kelly *et al.*, 1994: 31–2). These views are certainly understandable because, too often, postmodernism is only discussed at an epistemological level. This does not mean, however, that the issues identified by Kelly *et al.* are not being addressed by postmodernists. Hollway (1989), Stacey (1991) and Opie (1992), for example, have all looked at least some of these issues and all three are indebted to a lesser or greater extent to some version of postmodernism.

Conclusion

Researching on and in social work is currently quite a high profile activity (see Trinder in this volume). As she notes, feminist approaches to research have achieved a degree of influence. Given that social work research is often concerned with sensitive issues this chapter is offered as a limited contribution to thinking about researching such issues. It is also intended as a contribution to 'process' issues in relation to such research. What happens, how we feel, how we hear and read each other in the research encounter are vital issues which need ongoing discussion and debate.

Bibliography

Brannen, J. (1988) 'Research note: the study of sensitive subjects', *Sociological Review* 36(3): 552–63.

Cannon, S. (1989) 'Social research in stressful settings: difficulties for the sociologist studying the treatment of breast cancer', *Sociology of Health and Illness* 11(1): 62–77.

Cotterill, P. (1992) 'Interviewing women: Issues of friendship, vulnerability and power', *Women's Studies International Forum* 15(5/6): 593–608.

Fielding, N. (1993) 'Qualitative interviewing', in N. Gilbert (ed.) *Researching Social Life*, London: Sage.

Flax, J. (1990) *Thinking Fragments: Psychoanalysis, Feminism and Postmodernism in the Contemporary West*, Berkeley, CA: University of California Press Ltd.

—— (1993) *Disputed Subjects*, London: Routledge.

Gordon, L. (1986) 'Feminism and social control: the case of child abuse and neglect', in J. Mitchell and A. Oakley (eds) *What is Feminism?*, Oxford: Basil Blackwell.

—— (1989) *Heroes Of Their Own Lives*, London: Virago.

Holland, J. and Ramazanoglu, C. (1994) 'Coming to conclusions: power and interpretation in researching young women's sexuality', in M. Maynard and J. Purvis (eds) *Researching Women's Lives from a Feminist Perspective*, London: Taylor and Francis Ltd.

Hollway, W. (1989) *Subjectivity and Method in Psychology: Gender, Meaning and Science*, London: Sage.

Hooper, C-A. (1992) *Surviving Sexual Abuse*, London: Routledge.

Kelly, L., Burton, S. and Regan, L. (1994) 'Researching women's lives or studying women's oppression? Reflections on what constitutes feminist research', in M. Maynard and J. Purvis (eds) *Researching Women's Lives from a Feminist Perspective*, London: Taylor and Francis Ltd.

Laslet, B. and Rapoport, R. (1975) 'Collaborative interviewing and interactive research', *Journal of Marriage and the Family* 37: 968–77.

Lee, R.M. (1993) *Doing Research on Sensitive Topics*, London: Sage.

McRobbie, A. (1993) 'Feminism, postmodernism and the real me', *Theory, Culture and Society* 10(4): 127–42.

Mason, J. (1996) *Qualitative Researching*, London: Sage.

Maynard, M. (1994) 'Methods, practice and epistemology: the debate about feminism and research', in M. Maynard and J. Purvis, (eds) *Researching Women's Lives from a Feminist Perspective*, London: Taylor and Francis Ltd.

Nicholson, L. and Seidman, S. (1995) 'Introduction', in L. Nicholson and S. Seidman (eds) *Social Postmodernism*, Cambridge: Cambridge University Press.

Oakley, A. (1981) 'Interviewing women: a contradiction in terms', in H. Roberts (ed.) *Doing Feminist Research*, London: Routledge and Kegan Paul.

Opie, A. (1992) 'Qualitative research, appropriation of the "other" and empowerment', *Feminist Review* 40 (Spring): 53–69.

Philp, M. (1979) 'Notes on the form of knowledge in social work', *Sociological Review* 27(1): 83–111.

Rosenthal, G. (1990) 'The structure and "gestalt" of autobiographies and its methodological consequences', paper presented at X11th World Congress of Sociology, Madrid.

Sayers, J. (1991) 'Blinded by family feeling: child protection, feminism and countertransference', in P. Carter, T. Jeffs and M.K. Smith (eds) *Social Work and Social Welfare (Yearbook 3)*, Milton Keynes: Open University Press.

Segal, L. (1987) *Is the Future Female? Troubled Thoughts on Contemporary Feminism*, London: Virago.

Stacey, J. (1991) *Brave New Families*, New York: Basic Books.

Strauss, A. and Corbin, J. (1990) *Basics of Qualitative Research: Grounded Theory Procedures and Techniques*, London: Sage.

White, S. (1998) 'Analysing the content of social work: applying the lessons from qualitative research', in J. Cheetham and M.A. Kazi (eds) *The Working of Social Work*, London: Jessica Kingsley Publishers.

Chapter 8

Researching profeminist men's narratives

Participatory methodologies in a postmodern frame

Bob Pease

Introduction

Postmodern feminism has important implications for understanding and promoting change in men's lives, as well as women's lives. In recent years I have been exploring the implications of the relationship between postmodernism and feminism for emancipatory practice with men. I have argued elsewhere that a recognition of differences between men is central for understanding men's lives and for reconstructing men's subjectivities and practices (Pease, 1999a). I have also argued that the postmodern notion of the discursive production of multiple subjectivities has considerable potential for providing guidance to men about how their subjectivities and practices have been constituted and how they can be transformed (Pease, 1999b).

In this chapter I will outline some of the methodological and theoretical issues arising from doing research, within a postmodern frame, on the subjectivities and practices of profeminist men. Only a few heterosexual men have moved beyond personal change processes to search for a collective politics of gender among men and have recognised that they need to speak out against men's violence against women. Promoting collective responsibility among men to end men's violence is a central principle of many profeminist men's public practice. Profeminist men have been involved in the prevention of rape, speaking out against pornography, working to end men's violence in the home, opposing the military and organising in support of women's reproductive freedom. These attempts to develop a counter-sexist politics of heterosexual masculinity have been largely confined to middle-class men and there is much to be done to relate profeminism to the experiences of working-class men. Nevertheless, profeminism for men is one of the major forms of resistance to dominant masculinity.

I believe that men's subjectivity is crucial to the maintenance and reproduction of gender domination and hence to its change. The purpose of the research is thus to theorise men's subjectivities and practices to inform a profeminist men's practice in social work and to enact strategies that will, in themselves, promote the process of change. So the research is driven by practical concerns as well as by the imperatives of intellectual inquiry.

This project began with questions that have been a personal challenge in my search to understand my place as a white, heterosexual male social work educator who is committed to a profeminist position. What does it mean to be a profeminist man? What is the experience of endeavouring to live out a profeminist commitment? What do these experiences tell us about re-forming men's subjectivities and practices towards gender equality?

The nature of my research interests and commitment to praxis and change suggested a participatory approach to this exploration. As well, the implications of feminist critiques of mainstream masculinist research are, I believe, equally important for men's research with men.

Rethinking feminist standpoint theory

There are numerous debates about feminist approaches to research. Is feminist research primarily about how the topics are theorised and the findings analysed or is it also about methodology and how the research is done? Are there 'women's ways' of knowing as opposed to 'men's ways' of knowing? Can we talk about feminist methods and sexist methods of research, with methods inevitably flowing from epistemology? Can feminist research be done on men or is it only done with women? Can men do feminist research? In the context of this exploration, I have had to revisit these questions.

During the 1980s, three major methodological/epistemological emphases were claimed for feminist research:

1   a recognition of the open presence of the researcher as intrinsic to the process (Reinharz, 1983; Stanley and Wise, 1983);
2   a nonexploitative relationship between researcher and researched, based on collaborative cooperation and mutual

respect (Oakley, 1981; Glennon, 1983; Klein, 1983; Mies, 1983);

3   a transformation of the research process into one of 'conscientisation', a process of learning and critical self-reflection by participants (Mackinnon, 1982; Mies, 1983).

According to Halberg, the starting point for all feminist research is the critique of traditional social science as a 'male way of knowing' (1989: 4–5). Gilligan maintains that women are more inclined to link morality to responsibility and relationships and achieve power and prestige through caring for others. Men's development, by contrast, is said to be linked with fairness, rights and rules and they forge their identities in relation to the external world (1982: 5–23) and their modes of knowing are based on such ontology.

For Belenky et al., the masculine way of knowing is equated with 'objectivity, science and the scientific method in its emphasis on manipulation, control and distance from the objects of study'. Women, by contrast, are seen to adopt a more subjectivist position on knowing, distrusting logic, analysis and abstraction. They favour 'learning through direct experience or personal involvement with the objects of study' and are more drawn to knowledge that emerges from direct experience (1986: 71–4).

What do we gain by the notion that women and men think in different voices? Following Eisenstein, I would suggest that the association of masculinity with objectivity and science denotes a 'false universalism', based solely on biology and applicable to all men regardless of their theoretical position (1984: 132). I thus reject suggestions that men and women have *intrinsically* different ways of knowing which leads me to a critical review of the feminist epistemological approach known as feminist standpoint theory.

Many currents in feminism attempt to theorise grounds for trusting the vantage points of the oppressed and argue that there is good reason to believe that vision is better from below (Haraway, 1988: 583). Theorising from experience is juxtaposed to the notion that objectivity and distance are the best stances from which to generate knowledge. Instead, it is argued that 'the oppressed can see with clarity not only their own position but also that of the oppressor/privileged and indeed the shape of social systems as a whole' (Frankenberg, 1993: 8). Thus, feminist standpoint theory asserts that to start from women's experiences decreases the partiality and distortion of our images of nature and social relations.

For Swigonski, a standpoint involves 'a level of awareness about an individual's social location, from which certain features of reality come into prominence and from which others are obscured' (1994: 390). According to her, a researcher's standpoint 'emerges from one's social position with respect to gender, culture, colour, ethnicity, class and sexual orientation and the way in which these factors interact and affect one's everyday world'. Researchers are required to reflect upon the implications of their social position for both their motives for undertaking the research and the consequences for the conduct of their research (Swigonski, 1993: 172, 179).

In this version of standpoint theory, 'the less powerful members of society experience a different reality as a consequence of their oppression' and they must also understand the worldview of the dominant group to survive, resulting in their being able to attain a 'double vision'. They become aware of and sensitive to both their own perspective and the view of the dominant group which can enable them to gain 'a more complete view of social reality' (Swigonski, 1994: 390).

On the other hand, as Longino points out, 'women occupy many social locations in a racially and economically stratified society' (1993: 107). Should the standpoint theorist embrace these multiple and incompatible positions or endeavour to integrate the multiple perspectives into one? Maynard says that feminist standpoint theory lacks any real consideration of black feminist and lesbian feminist points of view and she convincingly argues that, rather than there being one standpoint, there are a range of different but equally valid ones (1994: 19–20).

Is just 'being' a woman a sufficient requirement to enable an accurate understanding of the world from a woman's standpoint? Swigonski argues that simply being a member of a marginalised group does not necessarily provide one with the vision that standpoint work requires. The standpoint of the less powerful group has to be developed (1993: 177). A standpoint that articulates women's 'true interests' has to be attained through political struggle.

Early formulations of standpoint theory were seen to articulate fundamentally different theoretical and political positions to that of feminist postmodernism (Harding, 1987) and some feminists engaging with postmodernism have positioned all standpoint theorists as operating within the Enlightenment metanarrative

(Flax, 1993: 142). However, I would argue here that there are a variety of standpoint theories that range from essentialist expressions and materialist analyses to postmodern variations. While earlier versions of standpoint theory did have an essentialising tendency, more recent interpretations have located women's experience in concrete, historical and discursive contexts. Furthermore, postmodern developments in standpoint theory have led to the rejection of a single female perspective and to the acknowledgement of a plurality of female standpoints (Grant, 1993: 91).

Hirschmann's (1992) distinction between feminist postmodernism and postmodern feminism is also useful in identifying points of convergence and conflict between the perspectives. While the tenets of feminist postmodernism are certainly in conflict with the emancipatory aims of standpoint epistemologies, I believe that postmodern feminism can use deconstruction to allow marginalised voices to be heard. Thus, I suggest that there is considerable overlap between recent versions of standpoint theory and postmodern feminisms that remain committed to emancipatory practice.

The possibility of profeminist men's standpoints

What are the implications of the debates about standpoint theory for profeminist male researchers? If where one 'stands' shapes what one can 'see' and how one can 'understand' it, from what standpoint can profeminist men study masculinity? If, as Harding argues, men also can create anti-sexist knowledge (1992: 178), is it possible to formulate a profeminist men's standpoint to study men and masculinities?

According to Morgan, when dominant groups research their own position in society, 'these considerations may be more in terms of justifications than in terms of critical analysis [and] their investigations may always be suspect' (1992: 29). He goes on to raise questions about the extent to which it is possible for men to develop those forms of self-knowledge which will inevitably lead to the erosion of male power and privileges (ibid.: 37).

If, however, men are seen to be locked into an ontological position within patriarchy, what space is left for us to explore our own masculinity? While we cannot individually or as a group 'escape' our material position in the social structure, I think that we *can* change our ideological and discursive position. The advantage of the notion of standpoint is that it relates to both structural location as well as the discursive construction of subjectivity, allowing us to distinguish between 'men's standpoint' and 'profeminist men's standpoint'. Following Frankenberg, I recognise that there is a substantial difference between the self-conscious engagements of oppressed groups with their own positioning and the self-conscious and self-critical engagement with a dominant position in the gender order (1993: 265). Nevertheless, I still believe that it is possible for men to change their subjectivities and practices to constitute a profeminist men's standpoint.

The process of change is itself a requirement in formulating a profeminist men's standpoint. Men have to change their vantage point if they want to see the world from a different position and this entails more than just a theoretical shift. It also requires men to actively engage in profeminist struggles in both the private and public arenas, translating in the possibility of a change towards more equal gender positionings.

There is feminist support for the view that it is possible for some men to change in the ways I have outlined and thus escape biological and structural determinism. Harding argues that men can make important contributions to feminist research and she does not believe that the ability or the willingness to contribute to feminist understanding are sex linked traits (1987: 10–11). Men can learn to see the world from the perspective of experiences and lives that are not their own and can thus generate knowledge from the perspective of women's lives. If women are not the sole generators of feminist knowledge, men are obligated to contribute to feminist analyses and in doing so, they must learn to take responsibility for the position from which they speak (Harding, 1992: 183, 188).

While it is a premise of this chapter that men can contribute to feminist theoretical work, there is a danger that the dominance of men will begin to assert itself on feminist knowledge by theoretical justification as a right. I believe that the most appropriate stance for profeminist men to take is the following: to hear feminist critiques of patriarchy, to research men in light of feminist theoretical insights and developments in methodology, to understand the origins and dynamics of these critiques from 'within' and to make the results of this research available for dialogue and critique, as a basis for working in alliance with women against men's social dominance.

The basis of men's contribution to feminist knowledge (and to their struggles) will be from our specific situation. Men have access to some areas of male behaviour and thought that women do not have (Harding, 1987: 11–12). In this sense, women cannot know the 'content of the deliberate strategies that men and male dominated institutions use to maintain their power' (Kelly *et al.*, 1994: 33). When men do research on men, it potentially enables the reader to eavesdrop on privileged consciousness and it reveals how men construct themselves in a dominant position.

On the other hand, there are further dangers when men engage with feminist issues. Reinharz is appropriately concerned that feminist scholarship is sometimes taken more seriously when men discuss it than when women do (1992: 16). Morgan has also pointed to the danger of men becoming so successful at deploying feminist methods, that they may attract research funding, set up centres and organise journals (1992: 183). Such dangers indeed exist but given that men value masculine authority more highly, they *should* use it to resocialise men (Harding, 1987: 12).

In light of the above, while men can support feminism, we cannot be feminists because we do not have women's experience. I prefer Wadsworth and Hargreaves' premise that men can do *profeminist* research if they can fulfil certain conditions, including making their work accountable to a critical reference group of women who will determine whether it meets their interests and addresses their problems (1993: 5).

This is not to argue, however, that feminism should set the agenda for men's research. Men have to take responsibility for the questions that emerge in their explanations of men and masculinity. While I would agree that some form of accountability by men to women is essential in researching masculinity, this does not involve the relinquishing of responsibility for determining the direction of the research. Making those to whom we are accountable arbiters of practice and research would, yet again, take away responsibility from men. This process of accountability must involve dialogue with women.

Participatory approaches to research

What, then, are the implications of the preceding discussion for the development of a methodology for this research? While it is generally accepted that men cannot do feminist research, they are encouraged to evolve approaches based on feminist standpoint epistemology to research men's lives and, in so doing, they must develop 'their own standards, directions, meanings, space and name for what it is they are doing' (Kremer, 1990: 466). Wadsworth and Hargreaves suggest that 'the methodological approaches of feminism will be relevant to men ... seeking to transform subordinating practice' (1993: 5), while Maguire also encourages men to use participatory research to uncover their own modes of domination of women (1987: 71).

Furthermore, experiential, participatory and emancipatory action research have histories and traditions that pre-date and go beyond feminism. Thus, while I do not claim that participatory action research methods are necessarily *more feminist* than other methods, they are more appropriate to the theoretical and activist concerns of my project. In addition to feminism, my exploration of participatory approaches to research draws upon emancipatory action research.

Emancipatory action research is at least partly based on a theoretical framework associated with Habermas' (1972) work, in that the participants' aim is to move from illusory beliefs that may be irrational and contradictory to a more enlightened understanding of the impact of social structures on their lives. Through the research process, people come to distinguish between what Habermas defines as instrumental and technical knowledge and critical knowledge which derives from the process of reflection and action.

From a postmodern position, Gore has criticised action research for failing to achieve its emancipatory intentions and for reproducing forms of domination because it functions within 'regimes of truth' (1993: 152–4). With Lather, however, I believe it is possible to reconcile emancipatory discourses and modernist strategies like consciousness-raising with a critical appropriation of important elements of postmodernism (1991: 1–2). They are not antithetical to each other as some postmodern critics suggest.

Within the participatory approach I have outlined, I have chosen three research methods to carry out the intentions of this research: consciousness-raising, collective memory-work and sociological intervention. All three methods involve group work, a precondition for participatory research and a preferred methodology for enacting the action component of the research process. Furthermore, the combination of the three methods provide a basis to bridge the gap between the individual and the social and between the subjective and the structural. Together, they avoid the danger of psychologising masculine subjectivities at the expense of structural change, while at the same time grounding the discussion of political strategies in the subjective realities of men's lives. I will examine the relevant methodological issues associated with each of these three methods and outline the process of operationalising them in the conduct of this research.

Consciousness-raising as research

Consciousness-raising is a method that reflects both my theoretical analysis and my commitment to activism. It enables participants to explore material about themselves in ways that are searching and insightful and while such a method focuses on the personal, it does not separate the exploration of subjectivity from the wider historical and political issues. Consciousness-raising is also a part of my biography and one of the processes through which I became aware of gender domination. As a method, it has a history, both in the contemporary women's movement and in the liberation struggles in Latin America.

Because feminist consciousness was not universal among women, one had to *become* a feminist (Bartky, 1975: 425–6). Hence, MacKinnon describes consciousness-raising as the 'quintessential expression' of feminism (1982: 535). The metaphor of 'raising' comes from the idea of 'bringing up' into consciousness experiences that have previously only been known at the unconscious level. It involves 'becoming aware at a conscious level, of things that we knew but had repressed' (Eisenstein, 1984: 35). This understanding and analysis are seen as first steps towards social change.

Against the postmodern critique that consciousness-raising is a modernist political project based on the 'meta-narrative' premise that people can come to recognise ideological and material domination and can struggle collectively towards egalitarian and socially just relations (Gore, 1993: 121–2), I argue with Janmohamed (1994) that it can be reconceptualised in postmodern terms. The process of consciousness-raising can encourage people to develop 'a relationship of non-identity with their own subject positions [which] requires an ejection of the introjected subject positions of dominant groups' (1994: 244–7). Thus, consciousness-raising becomes a process of assisting people to redefine their subject positions. McLaren and da Silva also position Paulo Freire's (1970) work on conscientisation within a postmodernist perspective (1993: 58) while Freire himself has recently acknowledged that his understanding of subjectivity, power and experience resembles some forms of poststructuralism (1993: x).

For my purposes, I find it useful to adopt Weedon's view of consciousness-raising, not as a method to discover one's 'true nature' but as 'a way of changing our subjectivity through positioning ourselves in alternative discourses which we produce together' (1987: 85). Thus, consciousness-raising plays a role in destabilising identity rather than creating a unified sense of self (Sawicki, 1991: 104), which means it challenges previously held conceptions of the self and creates the possibility for senses of the self to be reconstructed.

Having addressed these matters, I now face the issue of the implications of adopting a consciousness-raising process to work with members of a dominant group. Wineman used the concept of 'negative consciousness' to describe the process by which people become conscious of their oppressor roles and react against them. According to him, 'equal relations can be experienced as more rewarding than top down relations', which constitutes the positive foundation for negative consciousness. When one dehumanises people, one denies one's own capacity for emotional connectedness (1984: 187). Lichtenberg similarly argues that, once egalitarian relations are achieved, they can be as attractive to the dominator as they are to the subordinated (1988: 99). These notions provide the basis for a further discussion of anti-sexist consciousness-raising with men.

An initial response by men to the 'second wave' of the women's movement was to form consciousness-raising groups. Men's consciousness-raising groups have existed in Australia since the early 1970s, but these first groups had virtually disappeared by the early 1980s. Thus, when men began to return to the processes of consciousness-raising, they knew little of the existence of the earlier groups nor of what they had achieved or why they failed.

Many women were suspicious of men getting together in consciousness-raising groups, because they feared that this would be a reassertion of male power in the face of feminism. Such groups could be used as 'a resting place from which to continue oppression ... a way of avoiding confronting power over women by hiding with men' (Seidler, 1989: 173).

In spite of the dilemmas and challenges, anti-sexist conscious-ness-raising was seen by profeminist men as a way to understand their own sexist behaviour, to develop emotional support in other men and to encourage their anti-sexism. As such, these groups had and continue to have the potential to become an important part of profeminist practice by men.

We used consciousness-raising as a method to deal collectively with what it means to identify oneself as a profeminist man. We started by generating a series of questions. What are the basic problems that profeminist men face? What are the dilemmas and issues we grapple with as profeminist men? What accounts for these problems and dilemmas, given the gendered structure of society? Why is it that some men take up a profeminist subject position? What kind of subjectivities will support profeminist men's politics?

For many men who support feminism, there is confusion about how they are supposed to act. So, we began the process of identify-ing dilemmas associated with attempts at living out a profeminist commitment and arising within our own psyches, in personal relationships, in workplaces or connected to our political activism. No attempt was made to 'resolve' the dilemmas we identified; rather, this phase of the research sets the scene for the more in-depth exploration of the issues through memory-work and the further explication of them through dialogues with allies and opponents of profeminism.

The aim of this phase in the research process, following Vor-licky, was to analyse our position and develop 'a strategy for how [our] awareness of the difficult and contradictory position in relation to feminism can be made explicit in discourse and practice' (1990: 277). This necessarily involved an interrogation of our masculinity and a questioning of the privileges that are afforded to us by our gender.

The men in this study were thus involved in a process of re-forming their subjectivities and their practices in the wake of feminist critique and challenge. Through the conversations recorded in my research, these men revealed what it means for them to be profeminist. They tell us something about the personal and political implications of being a profeminist man at this historical moment, thus demonstrating that non-patriarchal subjectivities are available to men. These subjectivities, however, involve dilemmas and contradictions, for they are formed out of conflicting discourses and practices.

Anti-patriarchal consciousness-raising is one method for men to articulate and address these dilemmas and, through this, further re-form their subjectivities and practices by positioning themselves alternatively in new discourses that they produce together. This process of changing men's subjectivities and practices contributes to the struggle for the transformation of gender relations.

Giddens has observed that men have been 'unable to construct a narrative of self that allows them to come to terms with an increasingly democratised and reordered sphere of personal life' (1992: 117). The stories that the men told to the group are stories in which they are attempting to do just this. As such, these stories also provide new narratives which in turn have the potential to influence future stories and future lives. These men are self-consciously living the changes in gender relations.

Collective memory-work

Memory-work is a method that builds upon, yet goes beyond consciousness-raising. The method was developed by Frigga Haug to gain greater understanding of the resistance to the dominant ideology at the level of the individual, as well as how women internalise dominant values and how their reactions are colonised by dominant patterns of thought (Haug, 1987: 60). Haug describes memory-work as 'a method for the unravelling of gender socialisa-tion' (ibid.: 13). Her argument is that it is essential to examine subjective memories if we want to discover anything about how people appropriate objective structures (Haug, 1992: 20).

By sharing and comparing memories from their own lives, Haug and her groups hope to uncover the workings of hegemonic ideology in their subjectivities. Her particular concern is with the ways in which people construct their identities through experiences that become subjectively significant to them. The premise is that everything we remember is a significant basis for the formation of identity (1987: 40–52).

By illustrating the ways in which people participate in their own socialisation, their potential to intervene in and change the world is expanded. By making conscious the way in which we have previously unconsciously interpreted the world, we are more able to develop resistance against this 'normality' (Haug, 1987: 60) and thus develop ways of subverting our own socialisation.

Memory-work is carried out by a group of co-researchers who choose a topic or theme to investigate. It involves at least three phases. First, written memories are produced according to certain rules. Individuals are asked to write a memory of a particular episode, action or event in the third person without any interpretation or explanation. Writing in the third person encourages description and avoids rationalisation.

Second, the written memories are collectively analysed. After writing the memories, the co-researchers meet to read and analyse them. Each group member expresses her opinions and ideas about the memories and looks for similarities, differences and cultural imperatives. Memories are compared and contrasted with each other and appraised and reappraised by both the writer and others in the group so that the common elements are identified. Members of the group thus collectively interpret, discuss and theorise the memories. It is through this process that new meanings are created.

Third, memories are reappraised and analysed in the context of a range of theories. This involves rewriting the memories following the collective theorising (Crawford *et al.*, 1992: 40–51).

Memory-work is an example of what McLaren and da Silva call 'remembering in a critical mode'; it becomes a form of counter-memory. The purpose of this critical mode of remembering is 'not only to understand the past but to understand it differently (1993: 73–5). By recounting histories of oppression, suffering and domination, those who occupy positions of dominance can find ways to recognise their privilege and form alliances with the oppressed.

Memory-work has much in common with narrative approaches to research. Profeminist men's narratives can be read as counter-narratives because they reveal that the narrators do not think, feel or act as they are supposed to. In this context, narrative analysis also becomes a form of consciousness-raising that has both 'therapeutic and transformational possibilities at the individual, familial and societal levels' (Gorman, 1993: 257).

Memory-work is also consistent with critical postmodern approaches to research in that it enables us to identify how subjectivities are constituted discursively out of contradictions within discourses (Shotter, 1993: 409). It further emphasises the partiality of subject positions and the potential for agency that arises out of challenges from alternative subject positionings (Stephensen *et al.*, 1995: 2).

We used the method to explore both men's socialisation into dominant attitudes and the development of resistances to the dominant ideology. These processes were explored through an examination of four themes: men's relationships with their fathers, men's relationships with their mothers, homophobia and objectification of women. (see Pease 1999c and Pease forthcoming, for accounts of two of these memory-work projects).

Memory-work enables men to reflect upon and shape their own experiences and, in so doing, it contributes to the formation of non-patriarchal subjectivities and practices. The memory-work recorded in this research reflects sons' experiences of family life and following Hearn, I argue that to reclaim our experience as sons, 'through the self recognition of sonhood' is to challenge patriarchal constructions of fatherhood and manhood (1987: 187). Naming ourselves as sons provides the basis for the formation of alternative non-patriarchal subjectivities by repositioning ourselves against the dominant mode of identity reproduction.

Reframing our childhood memories also enables us to reconnect with our emotional histories and enables a critical stocktaking (Jackson, 1990: 110). Remembering is not only an attempt 'to understand the past better but to understand it differently' and it enables us to challenge dominant social relations (McLaren and da Silva, 1993: 75–6).

The family is, however, only one of the sites that form men's subjectivities and practices; we learn how to become men from a wide range of social practices. Two of these social practices are homophobia and the sexual objectification.

In these memories, profeminist heterosexual men described their involvement in the reproduction of hierarchical modes of heterosexuality. Reporting these memories, the men disclosed moments in their lives when they either challenged or accommodated to the processes of the reproduction of sexual dominance. They spoke from the dominant position about what it means to repress experiences of intimacy with other men and what it means to objectify women's bodies. They responded to Stoltenberg's challenge to speak a form of 'revolutionary honesty' and to say: 'This is what I did' (1991: 9). When men share the memories and stories of their part in the reproduction of hierarchical heterosexuality, they are subverting the construction of dominant masculinities. Furthermore, they are engaging in a process of reconstructing their subjectivities and practices in the arena of sexual politics.

Through memory-work, we explored the emotional and psychological basis of our relationships with women and other men. It provided the possibility for us as men to examine the construction of our biographies as personal to us and yet also constructed out of the materials and practices outside our own experience (Davies, 1994: 83–4). Remembering in these ways enables us to enter into a dialogue with our past, and through this dialogue to open up possibilities to challenge dominant social relations (McLaren and da Silva, 1993: 75–6).

Sociological interventions in masculinity politics

Alain Touraine's sociological intervention, a participatory research method specifically designed for the study of social movements involves, as a main principle, work with a number of activists organised in groups (1977: 6–7). The objective is to create a research situation which would, in some way, represent the nature of the struggle the participants are involved in. Thus, the researcher forms groups of individuals, who are involved in and identify with a social movement with the aim of engaging in some form of self-analysis. The incentive for individuals to become involved in the intervention is an awareness of disharmony between the ideals of the movement and its organisational practices (Touraine, 1977: 142–53).

Touraine discusses the importance of having different, even opposing aspects of the struggle represented in the group so that the tensions and conflicts of the movement can be brought out. Interlocutors, who confront the group with alternative analyses, are brought in to prevent the group from centring in on itself. The interlocutors are other participants in the movement, situated at different levels and engaged in different activities from those of the research participants (ibid.: 159–62).

Confronting the group with both its partners and its opponents brings out the field of their struggle. Through the dialogues, the members of the group have to answer to interpretations that differ from their own and to modify the image they previously had of their opponents. Touraine notes that this enables participants to overcome their rationalisations, as actors are encouraged to look critically at their own ideologies. The dialogues that take place model the main components of the struggle and after the meeting with the interlocutors, the group reflects upon the encounter and analyses the action (Touraine, 1988: 94–5). The group works because it has to resolve the tensions between its experience and its ideology and between its own view of the situation and that of the interlocutors. The main work of the group is to analyse its own internal discussions. It is through analysing the nature of the struggle, that the intervention reveals to the participants their capacities for action (Touraine, 1977: 167, 216).

At the end of the intervention, the researcher is presented with a diversity of arguments, debates and conflicts, out of which he or she must develop a set of hypotheses which will account for these statements and they are put to the test in discussion with the group. The researcher then makes an interpretation of the struggles facing the social movement. Is it a social movement or not? What directions does the movement take? What are its main problems and its most important conflicts and choices? How can its evolution be defined? When the intervention is completed, the participants return to action, where they match the conclusions of the intervention with their new experiences. On the basis of these new experiences, they return to re-examine the issues with their internal problems and increase their capacity for action (Touraine, 1977: 181–205).

There were five meetings with interlocutors in this research project: three feminist women; a mythopoetic ritual men's group; a founder of a men's rights group; a radical profeminist man who believes that it is not in men's interests to change; and two gay activists from a gay and lesbian rights group.

Each of these encounters posed various challenges to profeminist men's politics. All of the dialogues were tape recorded and transcribed and summaries reported back to the group who then considered the implications for how profeminist men position themselves.

Our dialogue with the feminist women invited us to consider the ethical responsibilities of ensuring that our work was accountable to the women's movement. It encouraged us to consider whether as profeminist men we are in danger of giving up our power, rather than using it constructively for non-patriarchal purposes. It invited us to explore the importance of profeminist men becoming more culturally compatible to reach a wide range of men.

The mythopoetic men argued that profeminist men are moti-vated by guilt whereas they are motivated by pride as men. In their view, moral imperatives about why men should change will not work. They argued that men will only change by healing them-selves.

The founder of the men's rights group argued that feminists inappropriately blame men for all that is wrong in the world and that this involves a denial of responsibility. He also argued that feminism involves men disempowering themselves and that it increases distrust between men and women.

The radical profeminist man argued that patriarchy is in men's self-interests so it is not in men's interests to support gender equality. In his view, the only reasons for men to be profeminist are ethical reasons.

The gay men were concerned that a gay affirmative position by profeminist heterosexual men may undermine gay men's space to speak out and that alliances between gay men and others may restrict gay men's identity.

These dialogues with interlocutors represented a microcosm of wider debates about the limitations and potential of profeminist men's politics. I am interested in finding ways throughout the process of developing a profeminist men's politics, of working out how to position ourselves in relation to the wider men's movement and to address the mythopoetic and men's rights tendencies in the movement.

I am also interested in forming supportive and constructive working relationships with feminist women and gay men. The aim of developing these alliances is premised on the belief that it is important for profeminist heterosexual men to join with feminist women and progressive gay men if we hope to be able to restructure the social relations of gender.

Prior to the 1960s, women's movements allowed a supporting but subordinate role for men who shared feminist views, but since that time, most feminists developed more explicitly separatist strategies (Phillips, 1993: 147). While many feminists will continue to be sceptical about men's involvement with feminism, a shift in opinion is occurring that could open up possibilities for profeminist men and women to work together again within a broader feminist movement.

Segal has argued that feminists needed 'to accept that part of their struggle must involve an alliance with men to transform the social inequalities' and she encouraged women to engage with men in progressive social movements of the left including labour parties, unions, community politics, anti-racist movements and the ecological movement (1987: 245–6). When marginalised groups pursue a separatist strategy, dominant groups are no longer pressured to re-assess their own attitudes and behaviour. Consequently, many feminists have argued that anti-sexist men can have a position in the feminist movement (hooks, 1992: 570–1).

Women will bring to this issue their own individual experiences of men, which will range from loving intimacy to violence and abuse (Luxton, 1993: 349). Thus, it is likely that women will continue to be divided between those who will work with men and those who will not. Furthermore, unless men have a committed anti-sexist stance and are responsive to feminist claims, they will not explore the potential to develop alliances with women to construct more socially just gender relations.

In acting as allies to women and gay men, profeminist men face a number of challenges. It has been recognised that when heterosexual men become involved with women's and gay campaigns, they 'often slip into authority positions' (Luxton, 1993: 352). There is a thin line between being a constructive ally and taking over another group's struggle. Even when men are sensitive to these issues, their involvement is more likely to be acknowledged and praised.

It is inevitable that allies will sometimes 'get it wrong'. They must overcome this fear by being willing to learn from women and gay men and committing themselves to challenge their own internalised domination. Straight white men will also have to accept that their offers of alliances will sometimes be rejected. This will at times lead them to be estranged from those they would want to support.

Making sense of profeminism for men

The theoretical lens that I use to make sense of profeminism for men can best be described as a postmodern feminist theory. From a postmodern feminist perspective, we learn masculinities through discursive frameworks and work out how to position ourselves 'correctly' as male (Davies, 1989: 13). Within these frameworks we are invited to accept or reject different subject positions and a sense of masculine identity that accompanies each of them. That is, each framework enables men to think of themselves as men in particular ways (Jackson, 1990: 286). Such a perspective enables us to identify that the supposedly fixed position between anatomical sexuality and gender stereotypes can be broken. We are therefore more able to legitimate behaviours that do not seem to derive from one's biological sex (Poovey, 1988: 59).

By conceiving of masculinities as discursive phenomena which compete with other discourses for the allegiance of individual men, there is greater potential for provoking inner change in men than the humanist notion of masculinity as an essence. The multiplicity of discourses lead to internal conflicts and contradictions for men opening up the possibilities for change.

The dominant discursive frameworks of masculinity are patriarchal but I maintain that men can reposition themselves subjectively in relation to patriarchal discourses and through evolving profeminist subjectivities and practices can resist succumbing to such masculinities.

In articulating a postmodern feminist framework and adapting it to explore the formation of profeminist subjectivities and practices among men, I have tried to provide a new language with which to understand the process of change for men, a language which enables us to ask new questions providing new insights into men's potential to change.

Postmodern feminism also provides us with a way of understanding those men who do depart from patriarchal subject positions. Self-identifying profeminist men are one such group of men. A profeminist commitment among men represents a major form of resistance to dominant masculinity. Profeminist practices by men challenge the standards of identity that give men status in patriarchal discourse and allow identification of alternative subject positions for men to take up. Progressive, straight white men are one group of men who are rejecting hegemonic masculinity and whose lives and experiences may contribute to our understanding of the process of forming profeminist subjectivities and practices.

Conclusion

In this chapter, I have argued that it is possible for male researchers to construct a profeminist men's epistemological and methodological standpoint as a position from which to research men's subjectivities and practices. I have argued that this standpoint must acknowledge men's positioning within gender, race, sexuality and class relations. I have also outlined the importance of my participatory research design, in this case, a combination of consciousness-raising, memory-work and sociological intervention, as a way of researching and reforming profeminist subjectivities and practices among men.

Men's practice in social work can either reinforce or oppose masculinisation. Thus men in social work have a part to play in reducing or eliminating sexism. We need to construct a new agenda for profeminist practice with men in social work and I believe that the participatory research methods that I have outlined in this chapter can contribute to that agenda.

These participatory methods constitute more than a set of research tools to elicit counter-hegemonic narratives. They also represent profeminist pedagogical interventions and practical strategies to assist men to construct profeminist subjectivities and practices. Furthermore, they link the discursively produced subjectivities of men to the prefigurative practices of profeminist action.

Bibliography

Bartky, S. (1975) 'Toward a phenomenology of feminist consciousness', *Social Theory and Practice* 3(4), (Fall): 425–39.

Belenky, M., Clinchy, B., Goldberger, N. and Tarule, M. (1986) *Women's Ways of Knowing: The Development of Self, Voice and Mind*, New York: Basic Books.

Crawford, J., Kippax, S., Onyx, J., Gault, U. and Benton, P. (1992) *Emotion and Gender: Constructing Meaning from Memory*, London: Sage.

Davies, B. (1989) *Frogs and Snails and Feminist Tales*, Sydney: Allen and Unwin.

—— (1994) *Poststructuralist Theory and Classroom Practice*, Geelong: Deakin University Press.

Eisenstein, H. (1984) *Contemporary Feminist Thought*, London: Unwin.

Flax, J. (1993) *Disputed Subjects: Essays on Psychoanalysis, Politics and Philosophy*, New York: Routledge.

Frankenberg, R. (1993) *White Women, Race Matters: The Social Construction of Whiteness*, London: Routledge.

Freire, P. (1970) *Pedagogy of the Oppressed*, Hamondsworth: Penguin.

—— (1993) 'Foreword', in P. McLaren and P. Leonard (eds) *Paulo Freire: A Critical Encounter*, London: Routledge.

Giddens, A. (1992) *The Transformation of Intimacy*, Cambridge: Polity Press.

Gilligan, C. (1982) *In a Different Voice: Psychological Theory and Women's Development*, Cambridge, MA: Harvard University Press.

Glennon, L. (1983) 'Synthesism: a case of feminist methodology', in G. Morgan (ed.) *Beyond Method: Strategies for Social Research*, London: Sage.

Gore, J. (1993) *The Struggle for Pedagogies*, New York: Routledge.

Gorman, J. (1993) 'Postmodernism and the conduct of inquiry in social work', *Affilia* 8(3), Fall: 247–64.

Grant, J. (1993) *Fundamental Feminism: Contesting the Core Concepts of Feminist Theory*, New York: Routledge.

Habermas, J. (1972) *Knowledge and Human Interest*, Boston: Beacon Press.

Halberg, M. (1989) 'Feminist epistemology: an impossible project?', *Radical Philosophy* 53(Autumn): 3–7.

Haraway, D. (1988) 'Situated knowledges: the science question in feminism and the privilege of partial perspectives', *Feminist Studies*, 14(3), Fall: 575–99.

Harding, S. (1987) 'Is there a feminist method?', in S. Harding (ed.) *Feminism and Methodology: Social Science Issues*, Bloomington: Indiana University Press.

—— (1992) 'Subjectivity, experience and knowledge: an epistemology from/for rainbow coalition politics', *Development and Change* 23(3): 175–93.

Haug, F. (1987) *Female Sexualisation: A Collective Work of Memory*, London: Verso.

—— (1992) *Beyond Female Masochism: Memory-Work and Politics*, London: Verso.

Hearn, J. (1987) *The Gender of Oppression: Men, Masculinity and the Critique of Marxism*, Sussex: Wheatsheath.

—— (1992) *Men in the Public Eye*, London: Routledge.

Hirschmann, N. (1992) *Rethinking Obligation: A Feminist Method for Political Theory*, Ithaca, NY: Cornell University Press.

hooks, b. (1992) *Black Looks: Race and Representation*, Boston: South End Press.

Jackson, D. (1990) *Unmasking Masculinity: A Critical Biography*, London: Unwin Hyman.

Janmohamed, A. (1994) 'Some implications of Paulo Freire's border pedagogy', in H. Giroux and P. McLaren (eds) *Between Borders: Pedagogy and the Politics of Cultural Studies*, New York: Routledge.

Kelly, L., Burton, S. and Regan, L. (1994) 'Researching women's lives or studying women's oppression? Reflections on what constitutes feminist research', in M. Maynard and J. Purvis (eds) *Researching Women's Lives From a Feminist Perspective*, London: Taylor and Francis.

Klein, R. (1983) 'How do we do what we want to do?: Thoughts about feminist methodology', in G. Bowles and R. Klein (eds) *Theories of Women's Studies*, London: Routledge and Kegan Paul.

Kremer, B. (1990) 'Learning to say no: keeping feminist research for ourselves', *Women's Studies International Forum* 13(5): 463–7.

Lather, P. (1991) *Getting Smart: Feminist Research and Pedagogy With/In The Postmodern*, New York: Routledge.

Lichtenberg, P. (1988) *Getting Even: The Equalising Law of Relationship*, Lanham: University Press of America.

Longino, H. (1993) 'Subjects, power and knowledge: description and prescription in feminist philosophies of science', in L. Alcoff and E. Potter (eds) *Feminist Epistemologies*, New York: Routledge.

Luxton, M. (1993) 'Dreams and dilemmas: feminist musings on the "man question"', in T. Haddad (ed.) *Men and Masculinities: A Critical Anthology*, Toronto: Canadian Scholar's Press.

Mackinnon, K. (1982) 'Feminism, Marxism, method and the State: an agenda for theory', *Signs: Journal of Women, Culture and Society* 7(3), Spring: 515–44.

McLaren, P. and da Silva, T. (1993) 'Decentering pedagogy: critical literacy, resistance and the politics of memory', in P. McLaren and P. Leonard (eds) *Paulo Freire: A Critical Encounter*, London: Routledge.

Maguire, P. (1987) *Doing Participatory Research*, Amherst: Centre for International Education, University of Massachusetts.

Maynard, M. (1994) 'Methods, practice and epistemology: the debate about feminism and research', in M. Maynard and J. Purvis (eds) *Researching Women's Lives From a Feminist Perspective*, London: Taylor and Francis.

Mies, M. (1983) 'Towards a methodology for feminist research', in G. Bowles and R. Klein (eds) *Theories of Women's Studies*, Boston: Routledge and Kegan Paul.

Morgan, G. (ed.) (1992) *Discovering Men*, London: Routledge.

Oakley, A. (1981) 'Interviewing women: a contradiction in terms', in H. Roberts (ed.) *Doing Feminist Research*, London: Routledge and Kegan Paul.

Pease, B. (1999a) 'Deconstructing masculinity – reconstructing men', in B. Pease and J. Fook (eds) *Transforming Social Work Practice: Postmodern Critical Perspectives*, Sydney: Allen and Unwin.

—— (1999b) 'Profeminist subjectivities: Working on the contradictions', *Mattoid* (forthcoming).

—— (1999c) 'Reconstructing heterosexual subjectivities and practices with white middle-class men', *Race, Gender and Class* (forthcoming).

—— (forthcoming) 'Beyond the father wound: memory-work and the deconstruction of father–son relationships', *Australian and New Zealand Journal of Family Therapy*.

Phillips, A. (1993) *Democracy and Difference*, Cambridge: Polity Press.

Poovey, M. (1988) 'Feminism and deconstruction', *Feminist Studies* 14(1): 51–65.

Reinharz, S. (1983) 'Experiential analysis: a contribution to feminist research methodology', in G. Bowles and R. Duelli Klein (eds) *Theories of Women's Studies*, Boston: Routledge and Kegan Paul.

—— (1992) *Feminist Methods in Social Research*, New York: Oxford University Press.

Richardson, L. (1990) *Writing Strategies: Reaching Diverse Audiences*, Newbury Park: Sage.

Sawicki, J. (1991) *Disciplining Foucault: Feminism, Power and the Body*, New York: Routledge.

Segal, L. (1987) *Is The Future Female?: Troubled Thoughts on Contemporary Feminism*, London: Virago.

Seidler, V. (1989) *Rediscovering Masculinity: Reason, Language and Sexuality*, London: Routledge.

Shotter, J. (1993) *Cultural Politics of Everyday Life*, Buckingham: Open University Press.

Stanley, L. and Wise, S. (1983) *Breaking Out: Feminist Consciousness and Feminist Research*, London: Routledge and Kegan Paul.

Stephensen, N., Kippax, S. and Crawford, J. (1995) 'You and me and she: memory-work and the construction of self', unpublished manuscript, Macquarie University, Sydney.

Stoltenberg, J. (1991) 'A couple of things I've been meaning to say about really confronting male power', *Changing Man*, 22: 8–10.

Swigonski, M. (1993) 'Feminist standpoint theory and the questions of social work research', *Affilia* 8(2), Summer: 171–83.

—— (1994) 'The logic of feminist standpoint theory for social work research', *Social Work* 39(4), July: 387–93.

Touraine, A. (1977) *The Voice and the Eye: An Analysis of Social Movements*, Cambridge: Cambridge University Press.

—— (1988) *Return of the Actor*, Minneapolis: University of Minnesota Press.

Vorlicky, R. (1990) '(In)Visible alliances: conflicting "chronicles" of feminism', in J. Boone and M. Cadden (eds) *Engendering Men: The Question of Male Feminist Criticism*, New York: Routledge.

Wadsworth, Y. and Hargreaves, K. (1993) *What is Feminist Research?*, Melbourne: Action Research Issues Association.

Weedon, C. (1987) *Feminist Practice and Poststructuralist Theory*, Oxford: Basil Blackwell.

Wineman, S. (1984) *The Politics of Human Services*, Boston: South End Press.

Chapter 9

For ever beyond

Lindsey Napier

Introduction

'Why don't you teach about death and dying? You must know something about it'. I'm caught on the back foot, because I don't know what stops me, other than the thought that death and dying are not one and the same. Another invitation to explore is lost. I'd like to turn to a body, a body of expert knowledge, social work knowledge, and hand it over to the student. But my hunch is that 'the knowledge' is firmly in the sociologists' and the counsellors' grasp. The student isn't asking me to point her in the direction of the library yet again, however, I am sure of that. I do not have an adequate explanation. I feel like a small child, gazing through a window into a room filled with learned experts, sealed off, just like death itself used to be. Or maybe still is? Either I'll have to find a way into the room, or stay outside and gather up some questions.

I suggest she borrows *Ceremony of Innocence* (Carmichael, 1991) and *Continuing Bonds* (Klass *et al.*, 1996), telling her that she will discover gems of social work writing. After many readings, I tell her, I am still astounded by *Ceremony of Innocence*, a book which explores the personal and social purpose and value of tears. I am humbled by the author's courage in sharing her belief that she had maintained her effectiveness as a social worker in helping others to be healed, in part by maintaining contact with her own wound, developed from 'the pain of the uncomforted child'. Here is no distant, detached expert who in social work reaches for the outside knowledge base alone and coolly decides which stage of coming to terms with dying or getting over someone's death the person has reached. 'I had tried to let the world come through me rather than round me,' she said (1991: 2). Her authority is richer.

Given half a chance, I'd like to have spoken too about *Continuing Bonds*, which explores the 'continuing internal connection' the authors discovered both adults and children bereft of a child or a parent develop over time with the one who has died. Reading it restored me to sanity. I remember thinking: here is evidence that life and death, living and dying aren't so neatly divided. My stubborn refusal to accept the thesis of 'disengagement' is now respectable. I am tempted to suggest that she thinks about death and dying as integral to the work she is doing in her hospital placement – not particularly specialised. Is not loss the central concept? However, I do not suggest that she read any of the textbooks on social work in health care, and particularly not the paper describing my own modernist framework for such practice. That would really show I'm out of date and avoiding the question! In the current Australian context of managerialised health services, the certainties are different. More importantly, that framework has come to make me feel distant from the experience of illness and from an engagement with people who are ill and dying. Its shelf life is over.

I send her off. She is one of many who have given me openings to assist their learning. I am reminded of Mellor's claim that, while in 'late' or 'high' modernity, death remains sequestrated from the public space, it is no longer a taboo subject (Mellor, 1993). Strong feelings about both death and dying abound and are expressed. 'I'm scared someone will die on me' is a common observation of students considering a hospital placement. (Yet within social work, there is a paucity of writing by social workers about social work with people who are dying and with people affected by the imminent and actual death of someone important in their life. For as much as it is 'everyday' practice for many social workers, it is not what we choose to write about it.) Others want to learn how to do 'it'. A few are very keen to work in the area, often seeing it as an opportunity to do some 'real' counselling or to find out how to stop unnecessary deaths. 'Three of the boys I went to school with suicided in the last year; and I want to find out more. I want to work in the area'.

Others yet again want to know how to avoid 'it' at all costs. For them, 'it' often symbolises a huge mountain. Climbing it will be a supreme test of their own survival: for them it is a dangerous field of knowledge. What will happen to them if they get very close to someone who 'dies on them'? Will they be able to survive the sight of a dead person's body? For these students, death and being left behind are foreign worlds.

The association between dying, death and old age touches students in different ways: working with old people was for one student an experience to be resisted at all costs. 'I've worked in nursing homes, my job was to wash all the [living] bodies; I'm sure it gave me a clinical depression and I never want to have anything to do with that again. Young social workers should not work with sick and dying people.' 'I'm totally disinterested in doing a course on ageing: I don't want to contemplate death and decay. Get a life!'

These are inimitable invitations. Such expressions of sheer disgust are not surprising for many reasons. As Vincent points out, 'There is some force to the point of view that in contemporary Western society, our particular set of cultural values relegates the very old to the undesirable status of living dead' (1995: 84). Contemplating the ageing bodies of old people (most often women) with whom one has no relation, providing them with routinised care for little reward is understandably offputting, when a secure sense of identity is so closely tied to a young, taut, disciplined body (Featherstone, 1991).

To date I've failed these students. On the one hand, I have resisted offering a programme called 'Death and Dying' with separate and specialised knowledge, skills and values to be siphoned off from the rest of social work. On the other, I have been unable to resist entirely the idea that working with people who are dying takes special(ist) people. After all, there is a burgeoning literature for professionals on the subject. It has become the province of experts in hospice and palliative care work. There is also an aura surrounding 'difficult' death work. Particularly in relation to disaster work, it is sometimes conveyed that one is either cut out for it or not as if it really is a test of survival, distinguishing the strong from the weak. Can dying and death be so sealed off from living and life, so 'precious'? I have no certainties but I want answers to my student's question. As I explain, I do not have frameworks of certainty to guide me.

In this chapter I describe a modernist framework a colleague and I developed for social work in health services and my increasing disillusionment with it. I move to a beginning engagement with postmodern and feminist ideas. I am choosing death, dying and bereavement as the focus of my enquiry, thinking at the outset that death, being the most certain thing of all would test *par excellence* the rightful place of grand narratives. But I'd no sooner started than a wise friend observed, isn't death the greatest uncertainty, the greatest mystery of all, the moment of greatest aloneness? In the light of postmodern and feminist ideas, this is a beginning exploration, a tentative breaking of my silence and a scatter of fragments.

Certainty

By the time my colleague and I came to teach and write about health service social work ten years ago, Australian community health services, which had burgeoned for a few halcyon years in the 1970s, were struggling to maintain their independence and philosophy. Their focus had been twofold: to implement the de-institutionalisation policies of psychiatric hospitals, and to strengthen the existing network of early childhood and aged care services by providing health education, health promotion and 'holistic' responses to primary social health problems. The language of the day was the provision of multidisciplinary, comprehensive, appropriate, adequate and acceptable services. The idea that health services could involve communities in creating resources for health and a healthy environment – knowledge, networks and programmes, for instance – was taken up with passion by some community health social workers. The new public health, with its emphasis on participation and involvement, was on the international agenda.

At state level, where I worked, it distressed me to observe the tensions, at least in the city, across a divide of 'hospital' and 'community' social work as to what should be the purposes of social work in health. It seemed to me possible for social workers who worked 'preventatively' with local communities using community development strategies to share the same analysis of the causes of ill health and the same approach to practice as social workers in acute and rehabilitation hospital settings. I had an interest in finding ways for community-based and hospital social work to 'pull in the same direction' towards a social view of health. I was searching for my own grand narrative! The project was intended as benign; I was (and am) interested in having the social determinants of ill health recognised and did not imagine that in some hands, the adoption of such an approach risked objectifying people. I too did not dismiss the possibility of grand schemes of change (Williams, 1993: 62). I omitted to remember that I am a social worker from the generation which was persuaded of the concept of a 'holding environment' in which people do *their* work.

The data emerging about the associations between social and economic inequalities, differential health status and access to health services, reinforced what I already 'knew' from personal and professional experience. Health status was closely related to material and ideological circumstance. I was removed from the immediacy of people facing sudden or gradually dawning changes in their lives caused by life-threatening illness or life changing trauma, sudden or imminent death of a family member. I still felt intimately connected to the world of the acute hospital, however, and could vividly recall how patients' personal and social needs can all too easily be separated from and made secondary to the diagnosis and treatment of their symptoms.

I wasn't altogether removed, of course, and on occasion, in situations of unexpected or large-scale disaster – rail, air and flood disasters – became the 'front line' response to sudden traumatic death and its aftermath. Because these events were extraordinary, and required 'one-off' disaster responses, I separated them from the emerging grand theory for practice forming in my mind. For me, crisis theory and intervention belonged to just that – crises – which were unanticipated, large-scale and did not have to fit my analysis.

With my social policy colleague, I provided an overarching theory for practice in health (Napier and George, 1988). We assumed a socio-structural analysis, arguing that while systems approaches did not close off the freedom to locate the causes of illness (and therefore the solutions) in the social environment, improving people's access to health resources, health chances and capacity to recover from illness, had to be grounded in an under-standing of the social determinants of health problems. Untimely death was to be prevented. Premature death associated with social inequality was unfair. This was progressive social work.

While the systematic social distribution of health and illness could only be changed through social solutions, we thought that it was important for student social workers to realise that 'the big picture' was not only 'out there'. It was everywhere, especially in the patient. The sick person in hospital was to be understood in terms of how gender, class, race, ethnicity, income affected their access to health resources and their chances of becoming sick. It demanded that a social worker understand the social construction of threats to life and living. Attempted suicide amongst old people could be considered as felt alienation in response to devalued role and status in a society where they are marginalised. As McLeod asserted, 'It is hospital social work's capacity – as social work – to foster health, which makes it so valuable' (1995: 21).

This framework promised certainty. It was strong on analysis of the distribution of health and illness, on the ways in which health and illness are socially constructed, on the relations of power in which patients become enmeshed. It framed my thinking; I could insert myself logically and objectively, move between different levels of intervention, assess with some certainty, know what needed changing and improving and how, all with the same framework in my head. So far as working with people who were dying was concerned, it demanded that the worker recognise that, as Small observes, 'We are not all the same in the end ... death is not the great leveller' (1997: 202). Through acting on the social situation of the dying person however, things could be improved both for the dying and those around them. There is of course support for this approach (Pockett and Lord, 1998).

Our grand plan touched few. It did not start where the clients – social workers, student social workers, far less people, who were called patients – were at. It started with a framework of under-standing, for establishing what were the likely characteristics about a person in their social location, what needed to be known, and what this might mean in terms of their likely expectation of the health service, the way their experience might be officially understood and responded to, the resources they were likely to be able to command or to need. And while it focused attention on differential death rates and systematic inequalities of access to resources for dying people it did not ask what the categories imposed on them meant for them.

Competing certainties

In any case, so far as social work with people dying and those bereaved was concerned, there were and are other frameworks which apparently offer(ed) social workers greater and more immediate security and certainty for action. Stage theory is one; systems and crisis theories a second; attachment theory a third. In the absence of research, whether and how such theories are followed through 'in use' or simply espoused is unknown.

It is likely, however, that even in the light of reservations and limitations voiced (Germain, 1984; Kellehear, 1990) interpretations of the psychodynamic theory of stages proposed by Kubler Ross became as familiar to many social workers as to other health care personnel. Smith (1982) for instance, in one of the few books on the subject in the 1980s, endorsed the validity of this knowledge for practice. It may be that stage theory has come to form part of the conventional wisdom about dying in social work (see, for instance, Davidson and Foster, 1995; Lord and Pockett, 1998).

The idea that people who are dying follow a series of stages from denial through to anger, bargaining, sadness and finally reach acceptance presumably provides a lens through which the worker can 'assess' a person's stage of acceptance and be confident about the direction the work should take. It may promise a sense of authority, control and predictability for the worker when working with people faced with terminal illness. Certainly, it can offer the worker the opportunity for distance from the experience of the dying person, allowing though not expecting them to remain the detached expert.

There were other certainties on offer, particularly for work with bereaved people. Phases of mourning, identified in a study of the responses of London widows to their husbands' deaths, have been described by Murray Parkes (1972). They provide a sure way of predicting the states and accompanying feelings of bereaved people. Numbness, yearning, disorganisation and despair, reorganisation may not proceed in linear fashion, but they occur. The worker can observe, assess, evaluate, intervene. Order can be imposed on the experience.

For what is to be done is also clear. The bereaved have work to do, grief-work; and the social worker is there to assist them perform it. Like others, Smith produces 'good reasons' why and to what ends bereaved people must confront the task of grief (1982). The pain of loss is to be borne, the reality of death accepted, the relationship with the person relinquished, unfinished business completed and alternative relationships formed. In America, as Charmaz has pointed out fifteen years on, 'resolving grief becomes a test of self' (1997: 231). (This strikes a chord with students when they convey that someone 'dying on them' presents a test of survival.)

The social worker informed by an ecological systems approach can be no less certain about the purposes of work with bereaved people. It is to evaluate and help with people's perception of the illness or death, their coping skills and the adequacy and appropriateness of their supports (see, for example, Williams and Rice, 1990). In this world of death and dying the social worker is an expert, presumably an instrument of the theory, continuously self-aware, understanding of and therefore in control of her own feelings and responses to dying and bereavement. She also, in my mind, stands apart.

Death is present but preferably marking the final stage in an ongoing contact, when the relationship established allows the social worker to 'monitor the situation' (Badawi and Biamonti, 1990: 149), assess how grief-work is proceeding and whether professional intervention is needed for people to move on to the next phase or stage.

I can't dismiss this out of hand. Stabbing memories of my own professional practice remind me that it did seem helpful that I stayed 'apart'. Put simply, during weeks of intensive physical, mental and spiritual caring for someone who is dying, I think carers do need someone who is caring for them, someone who can be utterly sympathetic without becoming an integral part of the drama, someone who makes it their concern to see that the carers retain residues of strength to cope with all that will happen as soon as death occurs.

I am left uneasy, however. I know that Kubler Ross never considered that the results of her work should be generalised, and yet stage theory is still taken for granted wisdom. But surely no one developmental pathway can encompass diverse experience. Death itself may be greeted with equanimity, in anger or as a friend, for instance. From the point of view of postmodernism, adherence to such 'objectivity' and 'certainty', as Leonard points out, does lead to our 'determination to control or hide others "in their own interests"' (Leonard, 1996).

Subjectivity

For the moment I'll have to ask the expert, the person at the centre of it all to wait. (They must be used to that!) I remind myself that only fifteen years ago, Kellehear pointed out 'The role of the dying in the construction of their "trajectory" was not given much attention, since staff and family reactions were seen to be more important' (1984: 7) He proposed that

> A way out of the dilemmas just discussed may be found in an analysis of the 'Good Death'. The 'Good Death' is a set of culturally sanctioned and prescribed behaviours set in motion by the dying and designed to make death meaningful for as many concerned as possible.
>
> (ibid.: 8)

As well, I agree that it is crucial to hear what the categories ascribed to the person who is dying mean to them.

I am reminded of my aunt's refusing to be thought of as sick in the last months of her long life, 'There's nothing wrong with me; I'm not ill. I'm just very old', she would say. She knew she would not die of 'something'.

I want to consider myself first, however. Since in social work, I am exhorted to 'use myself', I had better be clear who is this changing and constant self. If reflexive self-consciousness means anything, I am required to realise what I know and what are the limits of that knowledge, for whom I can speak. So far I've tried to keep myself out, hesitant about the authority of informal knowledge. Perhaps it is unnecessary to maintain this dualism: what is the point?

I am not free of knowledge. It was not uncommon in my childhood home for my mother, a nurse, to be called out in the middle of the night to sit with a family at home while a family member was dying and later for her to go and 'lay out the body'. This service was doubtless rendered freely, like all the voluntary work she contributed; and I took it for granted that what she did was women's work. Doctors visited to decide whether death had taken place, ministers took funerals, nurses did the domestic, private work of preparing bodies for interment. Being around death was a normal part of life. Indeed, my whole life has been shaped by death, by the fact that my father died a few weeks after my birth. Like all human beings, I have made my own meanings of this event in my life. This is a continuous process, one which changes me as I live at different points in time.

He died, as a Royal Air Force pilot, in the service of his country, thus making my mother a 'respectable' widow. He was reported 'missing' and presumed, for official purposes, to have 'lost his life'. I learned that when an identity, the embodied person, is difficult to establish and not seen, it may be difficult to believe that the person is dead. I learned that there may be a difference between someone being 'officially' dead, and being dead to the people who 'lost' him. I have learned of the importance of information, of finding out, but also of how vastly different family members can be in terms of that 'need to know'. One cannot prescribe one pathway.

I learned that the deaths of thousands of men and women was a fair price for winning a war. What was important in public, save for one day each year, Remembrance Day, was to celebrate the victory, not grieve the dead. I am interested to think about whose interests are served by the chorus of silent voices. I learned that just as much as for those who did 'return' to wives and lovers and sisters and mothers – or to nobody – and go on to lead 'normal lives' as for those families who did not, survival and getting 'back to normal' and getting on with life depended on calling on the stoicism, independence and endurance routinely expected at that time.

I benefited from a thousand sweetnesses as the child of my mother, a war widow. I learned of kindnesses at Christmas. I learned of being especially looked out for by aunts and uncles and teachers and 'our' minister. I learned of the efforts of one of my kin to include war widows in the annual Cenotaph march. I observed the price of widowhood at that time in that small, family-focused community – essential membership of the community, but social marginalisation.

I learned when and with whom to stay silent or to talk. In childhood listening to stories about my father was happiness indeed, he really did exist! I also learned not to talk about the fact that he was dead, the circumstances surrounding his death and what it all meant for any of us. I have learned more recently about 'delayed grief' and how it may be unhelpful to open up past wounds, how it may be better to 'let things rest', how some things are too painful for words, that after all 'it is so long ago' and therefore better to celebrate the happier times. I've learned, in other words, that the ways in which we act and feel are deeply contextual.

Finally, I've learned that keeping death at bay has perhaps protected me too. There have been other more personal meanings for me in maintaining this separation – left me with a fragile sense of life, as if it had been sheer coincidence which of us deserved to live, which of us must die. This is the meaning I have made; the meaning changes over time.

What I know about, however, is not about facing death or dying; it is about the meanings I have conferred on another's death; it is privileged and partial.

Normality

Such knowledge may be worth nothing, however. It can certainly be diminished or dismissed; and I have till now 'agreed' to dismiss it unquestioningly. For a start, as a young social worker, I came to act on the knowledge or belief that I was out of step with the rest of my generation. I succumbed to the pressure to believe the oft repeated statement 'People of our generation don't have any experience of death', with the silencing implied. I didn't have the right knowledge, whatever that was. Second, it can be dismissed because it refers to a specific place and time. It is just one story. That is all it is, one changing version of one truth.

Contingency

If then everything is contextual, what can I take from such learning? There is some understanding of changing sources of authority which people who are dying may bestow or have bestowed on them around dying and death. I have described a particular historical, cultural and bodily context in which dying and death took place. It has resonance with Waiter's (1994) description of both traditional and modern cultures, where authority was shared between religion and medicine. 'His time has come'. 'She wasn't meant to live' were as common statements as 'Doctor says she hasn't long', for instance. Death was less hidden, less managed by hospitals and life assurance companies. People knew how to behave: curtains were shut out of respect for the dead, shops closed for the funeral. Stoicism ruled.

In postmodernity, dying increasingly takes a long time. It is less easy to hide dying and death away when body parts can be replaced, when new, modern treatments can extend life and hope and immortality is tamed. One can take one's own authority: 'I'll do it my way'. Social work becomes part of the project assisting people to construct and re-order their own life narratives and 'sense of self', a project somewhat different from 'coming to terms' with dying and death through a lens of fixed identity (Mellor and Shilling, 1993). This is the context where increasingly social workers speak of blurring the boundaries between social and spiritual work: the concern is often expressed as an interprofessional concern in a secularist world. Just as 'pastoral care becomes, in the first instance, the task of enabling the person to articulate, or perhaps discover, what it is they believe' (Waiter, 1997), social work exhorts itself not to ignore the spiritual dimension of holistic care. It is necessary, however, to place that understanding within a broader understanding of cultural diversity and 'self-consciousness': authority may be conferred on different 'players' by the dying person and those around them, depending on the culture, time, place and belief systems they inhabit. To social work may be accorded none.

Professional practice knowledge

A different source of knowledge for me comes from practising social work, in hospitals and health services. In hospitals life and death, living and dying can be constructed as separate spheres. Death as the outcome of medical intervention may be regarded as a medical failure and saving life a medical success – 'we win some and we lose some'.

When I reflect on those years of practice, I realise that I have created my own oppositional categories, labelling some knowledge as 'ordinary' and other as 'extraordinary'. I have come to place the knowledge gained from practice experience firmly within the extraordinary category, resisted identifying what is common and dismissing it. To do so, I realise, infers that some deaths are extraordinary and others quite the opposite. I construct the rail and air disaster situations as the most demanding experiences of working with death and its aftermath. It is certainly true that involvement in major disasters and the arguments that followed to argue for the creation and retention of a social work service at a city morgue and coroner's court were demanding. There may be good evidence for regarding such extraordinary events as producing 'extraordinary' knowledge but I now see it as unhelpful to dismiss the knowledge gained, knowledge which is quite common. I learned about the responsiveness of human service systems to immediate crisis; about their equally firm 'back to business as usual' approach after a very brief time. I learned about the need to manage tensions between colleagues' need for rest after long hours of assisting family members in viewing procedures with their reluctance to pace themselves in extended crisis situations.

To create such a dualism is also deeply objectifying of the people who died, both there and in so-called 'ordinary' circumstances. Death may come to few people in such terrible ways; but it is not for me to say which words and meanings anyone will confer on their dying. It keeps death as separate, separate from the apparently predictable, yet risky business I call life.

I recall three children, whose mother, their sole parent, a young woman, was dying in hospital, more than twenty years ago. I do not know the meanings these three children ascribed then or now to the drawn-out dying of their mother, the woman with whom I sat, because there was no one else. What was ordinary about that? I recall the body of a young woman in death, hardly an inch of her body untouched by the wounds and scratches of abuse and neglect. Yet before death, she had described herself and her situation as 'no worse than the next'. To her, she and her body were quite ordinary, however extraordinary her body looked to me.

Body work

In remembering these experiences, it is impossible to erase memories of bodies. I do not know, however, what attention social work writing pays to the body. In this 'separate' literature, living and dying people seem to be present; the embodied person, living and dead, is absent. Yet social workers are often called when only the body of a person remains. They prepare people to see and identify disfigured, mutilated and unmarked bodies. They listen to what embodied persons mean to those called to face the sudden death of a partner, child, parent, friend. They are often involved when bodies are fought over, or when the legal ownership is transferred to the coroner and from the next of kin. They are often there to assist families, partners or friends decide whether any of them will see the dead body of their family member. They may quietly find a way to assist a woman break cultural rules and see the body of her dead baby. They may organise the disposal of unwanted bodies, bodies of persons whom no one wants to know.

They know that the status and respect accorded to bodies vary, and that the same bodies may be accorded respect long after their death. They help find bodies: still born babies of women, for instance, buried communally in graveyards unknown to their mothers, may many years later be 'found', 'remembered', and accorded respect. They know that however 'attached' someone may have been to the dead person, they may, following death, have no entitlement to claim next of kin status and no entitlement to make arrangements for the burial of the body, or indeed, no entitlement to mourn. Social workers often involve themselves in changing such policies and practices. It is rare in social work to read about this relation of social work to the dead. It is limited to the exhortation to be aware of which bodies will have greater or more unmanageable impact on the worker's capacity to focus on the needs of the living. Becoming 'desensitised' to bodies is still a goal, of necessity separating us the living from them the dead. This enables the worker to focus on the survivors.

It needs to be said that the typical death is no longer that of a child; it is of an old person, who may already have lived through the social death of being old and 'unattractive'. Bringing old people out of their homes and 'homes' into the public gaze – for outings, 'treats', – invites shivers of rejection and horror by those whose bodies are still disciplined and firm. Is that what we are to become? Is it the decay and death of the body or old age that is being kept at bay?

Places for dying

Modern places of dying invite professional specialisation. There are great benefits of this. For some people it is wonderful to live out their last days in the security of pain and sickness being managed expertly. It is essential for social work to be there and articulate the expert social work task (see Oliviere et al., 1998 for an important contribution in relation to palliative care). It is also helpful to name what is transferable to other contexts (Quinn, 1998). If the worlds of living and dying are not separate then all the usual things that happen in families are less private, less sealed off.

With increasing privatisation of responsibility for living and dying, increasing control over length of stay in hospital by health insurance companies, the rapid transition of the hospital to be a place of acute, surgical procedures and intensive diagnostic and medical management and the home as the expected place of convalescence, it is hard to imagine that many will be able to afford the ultimate postmodern dying experience described by Small (1997). As resources in publicly funded hospitals diminish, social workers in hospitals, and increasingly those who work in hospices, paint a different picture of the levels of luxury and choice available to people who are dying. More than once the comment has been made in relation to the retention or closure of palliative care units, 'Why should some have better treatment than others? We all have to die'. Death is always politically and historically contingent.

Beyond my grasp?

I am in my own room now and would invite another conversation with the student. I would ask her what she learned about dying and death when she was a child, when and how she became aware of them as facts of daily life. I am thinking that when one can speak about experience and not label it as abnormal, there's a chance to be fascinated about difference. Suddenly the idea of death education has meaning for me; it makes sense to bring death in from the cold, and out from the walls of the hospice and hospital. It allows us as social workers to consider whose deaths, and whose lives, are more highly valued than others.

So far as caring for people who are dying is concerned, I'd say to her it calls for open minds and prodigious leaps of the imagination. I'd suggest that in this matter we are all learners, since I think dying is both part of life and something neither she nor I have experienced. By the time either of us has first-hand knowledge (of that encounter) and has found the answer, it will be too late. The knowledge is forever beyond our grasp. I hope that is enough to start a conversation.

Bibliography

Badawi, M. and Biamonti, B. (eds) (1990) *Social Work Practice in Health Care*, London: Woodhead Faulkner.

Carmichael, K. (1991) *Ceremony of Innocence: Tears, Power and Protest*, Basingstoke: Macmillan.

Charmaz, K. (1997) 'Grief and loss of self', in K. Charmaz, G. Howarth and A. Kellehear (eds) *The Unknown Country: Death in Australia, Britain and the USA*, Basingstoke: Macmillan.

Davidson, K.W. and Foster, Z. (1995) 'Social work with dying and bereaved clients: helping the workers', *Social Work in Health Care* 21(4): 1–16.

Featherstone, M. (1991) 'The body in consumer culture', in M. Featherstone, M. Hepworth and B.S. Turner (eds) *The Body*, London: Sage.

Germain, C.B. (1984) *Social Work Practice in Health Care. An Ecological Perspective*, New York: Free Press.

Kellehear, A. (1984) 'The sociology of death and dying: an overview', *Australian Social Work* 37(3/4): 3–9.

—— (1990) *Dying of Cancer: The Final Year of Life*, Melbourne: Harwood Publishers.

Klass, D., Silverman, P. and Nickman, S. (eds) (1996) *Continuing Bonds: New Understandings of Grief*, Washington: Taylor and Francis.

Kubler-Ross, E. (1969) *On Death and Dying*, New York: Macmillan.

Leonard, P. (1996) 'Three discourses on practice: a postmodern re-appraisal', *Journal of Sociology and Social Welfare* XXIII(2): 7–26.

Lord, B. and Pockett, R. (1998) 'Perceptions of social work intervention with bereaved clients: some implications for hospital social work practice', *Social Work in Health Care* 27(1): 51–66.

McLeod, E. (1995) 'The strategic importance of hospital social work', *Social Work and Social Science Review* 6(1): 19–31.

Mellor, P. (1993) 'Death in high modernity: the contemporary presence and absence of death', in D. Clark (ed.) *The Sociology of Death*, Oxford: Blackwell.

Mellor, P. and Shilling, C. (1993) 'Modernity, self-identity and the sequestration of death, *Sociology* 27(3): 411–31.

Napier, L. and George, J. (1988) 'Social work and health care', in R. Berreen, D. Grace, D. James and T. Vinson (eds) *Advances in Social Work and Welfare Education*, Sydney: Heads of Schools of Social Work in Australia, UNSW.

Oliviere, D., Hargreaves, R. and Monroe, B. (1998) *Good Practices in Palliative Care*, Aldershot: Ashgate/Arena.

Parkes, C.M. (1972) *Bereavement: Studies of Grief in Adult Life*, London: Tavistock.

Pockett, R. and Lord, B. (1998) 'Perceptions of social work intervention with bereaved clients: some implications for hospital social work practice', *Social Work in Health Care* 27(1): 51–66.

Quinn, A. (1998) 'Learning from palliative care: concepts to underpin the transfer of knowledge from specialist palliative care to mainstream social work settings', *Social Work Education* 17(1): 9–19.

Small, N. (1997) 'Death and difference', in D. Field, J. Hockey and N. Small (eds) *Death, Gender and Ethnicity*, London: Routledge.

Smith, C. (1982) *Social Work with the Dying and Bereaved*, Basingstoke: Macmillan.

Vincent, J.A. (1995) *Inequality and Old Age*, London: UCL Press.

Waiter, T. (1994) *The Revival of Death*, London: Routledge.

——. (1997) 'Secularisation', in C.M. Parkes, P. Laungani and B. Young (eds) *Death and Bereavement Across Cultures*, London: Routledge.

Williams, C.C. and Rice, D.G. (1990) 'The intensive care unit: social work intervention with the families of critically ill patients', in K.W. Davidson and S.S. Clarke (eds) *Social Work in Health Care*, Binghampton, NY: Haworth.

Williams, F. (1993) 'Postmodernism, feminism and the question of difference', in N. Parton (ed.) *Social Theory, Social Change and Social Work*, London: Routledge.

Chapter 10

Feminist postmodernism in the South African context[1]

Vivienne Bozalek

Introduction

> For all its talk of difference, plurality, heterogeneity, postmodern
> theory often operates with quite rigid binary oppositions, with
> 'difference', 'plurality' and allied terms lined up bravely on one
> side of the theoretical fence as unequivocally positive, and what-
> ever their antithesis might be (unity, identity, totality, univer-
> sality) ranged balefully on the other.
>
> (Eagleton, 1996, cited in Sim, 1998: 25)

The historic release of Nelson Mandela and the first ever democratic
elections in 1994 have heralded significant changes in South Africa
during the past decade. Since then, efforts have been made to
dismantle the divide and rule policy of the apartheid regime and
construct a new policy. The justification for the apartheid policy in
South Africa was based upon notions of difference, specifically in
terms of 'race' and 'culture' and this is why, during the reconstruc-
tion period, there has been a foregrounding of unity, equality and
universality. This has been in direct contrast to feminist postmodernist ideas in the North in the same period, which have emphasised the notion of difference in the place of equality. In the
apartheid era, the notion of difference has had lethal consequences
for the majority of the South African population, who were
construed as different and in need of 'separate development'
(apartheid). In this context, difference as a concept has therefore had
a contaminated past. Is it possible, as Rosi Braidotti (1997) has
suggested, to 'cleanse' the notion of difference so that it could be
made useful in our situation? In this chapter, I make an attempt to

answer this question by looking at the problems and possibilities that feminist postmodernism offers in the South African context. I conclude that although difference in the apartheid context has been used to justify disqualifying, objectifying and marginalising the majority of the population, and therefore as tainted, the concept can be 'cleansed' and that a feminist postmodern lens would be valuable for analysis of past and present social work policy and practice in South Africa.

South African social work

Some social work writers have argued that social policy cannot be analysed from a postmodern perspective since its focus is on macro issues which postmodernism rejects (e.g. critique of Howe (1994) and Parton's (1994) use of postmodernism in social policy by Smith and White (1997)). I would not agree with this and prefer Fraser and Nicholson's (1990: 34) argument that postmodern feminists need not abandon large theoretical tools or analyses of societal macrostructures, but that these analyses must be explicitly historical and be situated within particular cultural and historical contexts. I have found particularly useful in analysing South African social policy, Nancy Fraser's (1989) analysis of the politics of needs interpretation through applying discourse analysis, showing how needs discourses are the products of political struggle over meaning. This text has provided a useful feminist postmodern critique of social work policy, particularly of the way in which women clients are positioned in the welfare system. Another illuminating text is that of Linda Gordon and Nancy Fraser's genealogy of the concept 'dependence' in demonstrating how certain groups of people such as single Black mothers are demonised and excluded in America. I have utilised these texts to deconstruct past and current post-apartheid social policy on child maintenance grants in South Africa from a feminist postmodern perspective (see Sunde and Bozalek, 1995; Bozalek, 1997; Naidoo and Bozalek, 1997).

South African welfare services have been premised upon social and political exclusion of the majority of its population, and this has been achieved through what O'Brien and Penna (1998: 206) have termed the 'race-ing' of its welfare services, resources and systems. This demonstrates the effects or consequences of empha-sising difference – the foundation upon which apartheid was built. O'Brien and Penna give a useful explanation of postmodern perspectives on citizenship which can be used in social policy analysis:

> Postmodern theory points to the 'decentring' of the social relations of welfare. Whilst social policy traditionally has served to represent a process of public incorporation and collective development, postmodernism points to the cultural fracturing of, and domination in, public and private life. Postmodernism shifts attention away from normative issues of defining universals, applying objective knowledge to planning and realising rational goals. Instead, it focuses on the multiple and uneven frameworks of power that sustain the fragmentation of political and institutional life and how these networks support definitions of what is 'universal', 'rational' and 'objective'. In this regard, postmodern perspectives challenge the rationality of traditional policy discourses and practices and contest their logics, conventions and norms.
>
> (ibid.: 201–2)

This is a fruitful reference point for discussing how difference was largely racialised and also gendered in South African social welfare policy. Social work in South Africa has largely been directed at the white group, with coloureds and Indians having been marginally included and Africans almost entirely excluded.[2] The dominant identity has been constructed and protected by othering and excluding the so-called 'others'.

The use of difference in South African welfare policy

Before 1948

In 1925 the Urban Areas Act provided for the sale of municipally produced 'Kaffir beer' the proceeds of which was proposed to finance African welfare, housing and recreation – in other words, the poor were to pay for their own services. Another justification for ignoring Black needs was that Africans were constructed as having their own traditional family system to provide for their welfare needs.

After the Anglo-Boer war at the beginning of this century, which was seen to have devastating consequences for the Boer population, the discourse of white poverty became prominent. Government relief schemes were initiated in response to this discourse and in 1932 the Carnegie Commission produced a report on the poor white problem. In 1936 at the National Conference on Social Welfare, Dominee Nicoll, in his opening address, said as justification for the focus on whites: 'It should be clear to everyone that we cannot do much to solve the Native question unless we first solve the Poor White problem' (Kotze, 1996). This discourse was institutionalised and had material implications in the Carnegie Report on Poverty and a Volkskongres held in 1934, resulting in the establishment of the Department of Welfare in 1937 to cater for the needs of poor whites. This led to the training of social workers at universities and the emergence of the profession of social work. The welfare system was a residual one, in which the individual was held responsible for his/her well-being with the state intervening as the last resort. However, other policies such as protected employment, low cost housing and free education were put in place to support whites. (Greater Johannesburg Welfare, Social Service and Development Forum's Submission to the Truth and Reconciliation Commission, 1998).

In the meantime, the dispossession of the indigenous people was being carried out by legislation which was enacted by the South African government prior to the apartheid era from 1948–93, but which was intensified once the Nationalists came into power in 1948. The 1913 Land Act reserved 90 per cent of land for white use and the Native Urban Areas Act of 1923 confined Africans to rural reserves, which later became homelands. This homelands policy designated ten small areas as homelands for Africans, who formed the majority of the population, resulting in widespread poverty and the inability of inhabitants to sustain subsistence farming. This led to men migrating mainly to the mines to search for work. Wives and children were left in the homelands to survive on the small amounts of money that the men sent back. It was illegal for women to follow their men to urban areas so they either starved in the homelands or illegally lived in men's hostels or informal settlements on the outskirts of the urban areas. Children were often cared for by family members or relations other than their biological parents, as their mothers also left home to seek employment as domestic workers, and schools were not available to them in rural areas so they were sent to relatives or boarding school.

The apartheid era – post-1948

From 1948, the restriction of movement was accelerated through the dominant ideology of separate development or apartheid. The following laws were passed which had implications for Black South African families: The Group Areas Act 41 of 1950; The Prevention of Illegal Squatting Act 52 of 1951; The Blacks Resettlement Act 19 of 1954.

These Acts had devastating consequences for Black South African families. Between 1960 and 1983 it was estimated that 3.5 million people were forcibly removed from their homes causing economic, physical and psychological suffering (Bundy, 1990: 8). Over twenty-five years this had the effect of not only removing the productive and physical assets of people, forcibly dispossessing households of land and cattle and relocating them into Bantustan homelands in rural areas and wastelands far from areas of work and community resources in the urban areas, but also cutting people off from their kin and community contacts and infrastructure. It is ironic to note that during this period of intentional dislocation of Black South African families, the Department of Welfare was eulogising 'the family', as evident in the following statement by the Department of Social Welfare during this period:

> Family life is one of the greatest heritages that civilisation has left us. There is no greater influence for character forming and spiritual strengthening. The family circle is the one place where the fundamental human relations are nurtured. It is the cradle of our deepest emotions and most highly prized traditions and of everything that we regard as noble and fine.
>
> (Department of Social Welfare, South Africa, 1950: 71)

If these were the state's sentiments about the family why were they condoning and reinforcing the above legislation which was tearing families apart? The answer is that only whites were constructed as constituting families.

Numerous discriminatory practices and legislation were justified by the discourse that it was in the best interests of Africans, especially women and children, to remain in the reserves. So for example, Harvey (1994: 36) reports that as a consequence of the Children's Act 31 of 1937, a family allowance scheme, later referred to as the State Maintenance Grant, was made available to whites, coloureds and Indians, with whites being paid double the allowance of the other groups.

African children were excluded under the pretext that their needs were being met in the 'tribal context' in the reserves. As I have previously indicated, the mission of the Department of Welfare, established in 1937 was to foreground white needs only, and the 'Poor White problem' that existed in the 1930s was largely eradicated through a well-developed and co-ordinated national socio-economic strategy (Mazibuko, 1996: 1). Although the authorities acknowledged that living conditions were not favourable for the coloured population, no attempt was made to improve them. The Indian population was constructed as an exogenous group and ignored on this basis (Harvey, 1994: 18). In 1945 it was reported that 10 per cent of white families, 45–50 per cent of Indian families, 50–60 per cent of coloured families and about 75 per cent of Black families earned so little that the wage-earner could not afford what had been termed a 'bare-minimum diet' (Committee for Social Security, Suid Afrika, 1945: 18, cited in Harvey, 1994: 33).

During the 1950s racial separation of state welfare services was instituted with the Departments of Bantu Administration and Coloured Affairs being set up to deal with African and coloured persons, respectively. The Department of Indian Affairs was initiated in 1961. Services were further divided by homelands governments setting up their own departments for welfare services. Voluntary organisations still exercised some choice with regard to whom they served, although there was never a strong service for Black clientele. This position changed with Circular 29 of 1966, issued by the then Department of Social Welfare and Pensions (Greater Johannesburg Welfare, Social Service and Development Forum's Submission to the Truth and Reconciliation Commission, 1998: 3). This Circular reminded welfare organisations of the state's policy that each population group should serve its own community in the sphere of welfare, and admonished welfare organisations that the practice of maintaining multi-racial organisations and having representatives of different races at council and committee meetings was contrary to this policy. The following reasoning which was offered in the Circular for this policy, serves to demonstrate how practices of racism became normalised through state policy documents:

a. Meetings of White bodies are held in White areas, usually at well-known venues where non-Whites do not normally go, and there is every likelihood that this will give rise to talk, criticism, friction and so on.

b. Experience has shown that one or two non-Whites at a meeting of Whites are far less effective than when the position is reversed, because the non-Whites, being a minority group, are over-shadowed and therefore do not make a fruitful contribution unconstrainedly.

c. In the case of some non-Whites we have to a certain extent to deal with their need for recognition of status and encouragement towards independence, a need which is not gratified when non-White delegates, as outsiders, have to act in a larger White group.
(Republic of South Africa, Department of Social Welfare and Pensions (1966) Circular No. 29 of 166)

What is interesting to note here is the construction of the 'non-White' group as outside interlopers into the world of white privilege and as a minority, whereas it has always been the vast majority in the country. The reason given for exclusion of Black social workers in terms of the awkwardness of social situations at tea-breaks and meals imply that whites could not contemplate eating or drinking tea with their Black colleagues. This circular also demonstrates the patronising attitude towards all that were othered as 'non-White' whose 'status is to be recognised' and whose 'independence' has to be 'encouraged'. These justifications for racist policies in non-state welfare organisation sector now seem ludicrous, but what is alarming is that this was regarded as 'rational' discourse at the time. This piece of policy material demonstrates the important linguistic devices that were used to portray all those who did not fit into the favoured 'white' category as abnormal. Policy documents such as these give an indication of the scaffolding upon which apartheid practices were built. This document serves as an illustration of how the South African state was able to control knowledge, meaning and practice and exercise power through disciplinary and professional institutions such as social work.

It is documents such as these which make one understand how the notion of difference has an ominous tone for South Africans, as overtly brutal and racist legislative policy became normalised in the apartheid era. At this time, whites were called upon by the state not to 'mix politics with social work' (Greater Johannesburg Welfare, Social Service and Development Forum's Submission to the Truth and Reconciliation Commission, 1998: 4). It has only been at the Truth and Reconciliation hearings that previously privileged (white) social workers have begun to review their own complicity in the marginalisation of the Black majority.

As a reaction to the enforced particularities and use of notions such as pluralism by the divide and rule apartheid state policy, South Africa seems to be at this point in time, one of the few countries in the world in which a modern emancipatory project of universalism, unity and cohesive struggle is embraced by the majority who have been a marginal group. In 1994, South Africa held its first historic democratic elections and now has a new Constitution which emphasises non-sexism, non-racism as opposed to anti-racism and anti-sexism – terms which emphasise difference in a more stark way. The founding provisions of the Constitution (1996) are the following:

> The Republic of South Africa is one, sovereign, democratic state founded on the following values:
>
> a) The safeguarding of basic human rights and freedoms.
> b) Non-racialism and non-sexism.
> c) Universal adult suffrage, a national common voters roll, regular elections and a multi-party system of democratic government to ensure accountability, responsiveness and openness.
>
> (Republic of South Africa (1996) *The Constitution*, Republic of South Africa Act 108, Wynberg, Constitutional Assembly: 3)

There has also since 1994 been much rhetoric about 'the Rainbow nation', where differences are implied but homogenised, as power is elided within the concept of a 'Rainbow nation', making the groups encompassed in it equivalent, rather than positioned in relations of power and subjugation. This romantic notion of the Rainbow nation is a strong reaction to the racialised hierarchies of the apartheid era, but the inter-ethnic and political tensions which have resulted in large-scale murders between groups as a result of apartheid, but after its demise, have posed a strong contrast to the romanticism of the 'Rainbow nation'. The 'Rainbow nation' is problematic in that it could result in a premature glossing over of apartheid atrocities and the consequences thereof for differently situated groups in South Africa. Instead of the symmetrical pluralism of the 'Rainbow nation' we need a concept which conveys the asymmetrical positioning of markers of difference in South Africa.

The notion of an African renaissance has recently received much attention in South Africa, and is advocated particularly by the Deputy President of South Africa, Thabo Mbeki, among others. Mbeki (1998: 30) envisages the African renaissance as reclaiming the creativity and history of Africa and thus restoring an African cultural identity – to reclaim the status of being fully human. While this notion is important in affirming ties within Africa and building a sense of pride and dignity to the previously subjugated and colonised, Africans are seen as a distinct cultural and ethnic group, which precludes fluidity and relationality. It could be construed as a fixed unitary complete position where Africanness is essentialised and it takes on the guise of the truth as opposed to eurocentrism. This is another totalising theory – another way of legitimising certain statements and denying others authority. This also brings us back to the question of whether it is only the oppressed who can generate knowledge – can an understanding of oppression only come out of the experience of oppression? In my view there is a real danger of equating certain types of experience with 'the truth' and with valid knowledge. The notion of contradictory identities and contradictory social locations which are shifting seems to be preferable. I tend to support Dennis Davis, a legal academic who observed the following in an address:

> The call for Africanisation is commendable where it is designed to promote a greater inclusivity and an engagement with the riches of the identity, culture and history of Africa. That we need to test previous assumptions and shibboleths in the light of an engagement with Africa is surely a major educational imperative. But this is not to be conflated with the view that the education system must be there to emphasise the unity of the nation, at the expense of group or local diversity.
>
> (Davis, 1998: 24)

The scarcity of texts on postmodernism in South Africa, and more particularly on feminist postmodernism may be an indication that this paradigm shift has not been considered relevant to the present South African situation. It is only in psychology that any texts have appeared. (Notably that of Levett *et al.*,1997, entitled *Culture, Power and Difference: Discourse Analysis in South Africa*, the contents of which were largely drawn from a discourse analytic workshop at the University of Cape Town in 1994.)

It is only recently in South African social work journals that articles which deal with feminism have appeared, and there has been no debate with regard to the turn to postmodernism within local social work circles. I have also recently attended two national social work conferences, one involving educational institutions and the other the state department, practitioners, policy-makers and academics, where little reference was given to postmodern analysis (one paper on the narrative approach to teaching) and where gender was included as an 'add on' approach. These omissions may perhaps be the result of the conservatism of South African social work, but the changing emphasis on unity and cohesion within South Africa may also have contributed towards this. The postmodern focus on difference and multiplicity may be regarded as a threat to the newfound cohesion which the so-called new Government of Unity has brought to South Africa. It is said in some circles that South Africa is one of the few countries in the world where the Communist Party has maintained its credibility. The African National Congress, as a humanist emancipatory movement, was led by an orientation towards totalising universal human emancipation and continues to uphold this ethos, in which other struggles such as the women's movement, workers, etc. are assimilated under the general project of the advancement of humanity.

Foucault's ideas of professions such as psychology and social work being institutions through which disciplinary power is exercised and through which individuals are controlled is particularly pertinent to the South African situation where social work has in some instances been used directly by the apartheid state to 'discipline and punish' dissidents and freedom fighters of the apartheid regime. For instance, when Shirley Gun, previously a social worker, but also an ANC cadre was detained with her seven-month-old baby who she was breastfeeding at the time, state social workers removed the baby from her to a place of safety in an attempt to punish her. This inhumane act caused severe distress for both mother and child.

In our social work curriculum, students are taught values of human dignity and self-determination and in the social work philosophy course notions such as personhood and 'brotherly love' (sic) are covered. I have also attended both national and international conferences on social work where the social control aspects of the profession are never referred to, and one has a sense of social work as a benevolent force, which is far removed from the image of social workers in working-class coloured townships in South Africa where children are threatened behave or 'the welfare' will come and get you. I believe that South African social work could benefit from feminist postmodern analyses of how the profession has been used as a means of social control.

Problems and potentials of feminist postmodern perspectives in the South African context

Sandra Harding (1990) has raised the question that if women have never been 'modern', how can we skip this phase and go straight into postmodernity? Women have never been regarded as moral agents and knowing subjects, and the project of feminism has been to transform women into moral agents and knowing subjects. When this may be a possibility, the rug is pulled from under their feet by postmodernists who question the very legitimacy of these notions. Feminist scholars from the South, in particular those concerned with issues of poverty, have tended to dismiss postmodernism as a luxury or indulgence that only Northern women with time and resources can afford to angst over (Parpart and Marchand, 1995; Burman, 1998). Nancy Hartsock (1996) is also critical of the contribution that postmodernism can make to feminism as she points out that both Enlightenment and postmodern perspectives have been produced by the same privileged group of people – Euro-American, masculine and racially as well as economically privileged. Sandra Harding also makes this point wondering why anything that is not produced in the North is not regarded as a legitimate knowledge. In the South African context, Lewis (1997) has argued that postcolonial theory has been developed by white academics in disciplines such as English or history – not conventionally politicised disciplines, that these academics are situated at the centre rather than at the margins and that the language they use is esoteric.

Hartsock maintains that postmodernism leads to nihilism or epistemological despair and denial of agency. She argues that we should instead use our 'marked subjectivities' to develop partial or situated knowledges which are located at a particular space and time. For Alcoff (1995: 442), if we were to follow Foucault and Derrida's views, an effective feminism could only be a negative one, deconstructing everything and refusing to construct anything. In the South African context where the present emphasis is on rebuilding the social fabric, this would not be an adequate stance to take.

It is not a postmodern strategy to outline courses of action or prescribe what should be done – Foucault argues that the role of the intellectual should be the destabilisation of the pretensions of other theories or the 'disturbance of people's mental habits' (Foucault, 1988: 285, cited in Ramazanoglu, 1993: 11). Postmodernists are also not comfortable with closure on issues and prefer to leave questions dangling and unanswered (Hirschmann and Di Stefano, 1996: 21). I think, however, that it would be necessary to assess in what way feminist postmodernism could be useful in the South African social work context. We need also to look at what would be appropriate intellectual spaces for work within this context.

Rather than focusing solely on the local in social work and social policy, as some postmodernists would advocate, we need transnational comparisons of similar communities and situations, intertwining the local and the global, e.g. tracing the history of Aid For Dependent Children (AFDC) and the new Temporary Assistance to Needy Families (TANF) in the United States and comparing this with the State Maintenance Grant and the new Child Support Benefit in South Africa and social security for single women in other countries. One could examine the global move from welfare to workfare and the surveillance by the state of women who are regarded as dependent. The structural adjustment programmes of the International Monetary Fund (IMF) and the World Bank and the current global economic crisis could provide the backdrop for this analysis. This would entail a politics which is based on multiple socially constructed identities, which is developed through local and specific forms of agency, but which relates transnationally to issues of globalisation. This is similar to Alcoff's suggestion, which is to insist on the non-essentialised status of gender, while using this position from which to act politically. Chandra Mohanty has termed this 'strategic essential-ism', where one works within inherited and oppressive discursive categories, shaped by contextually specific relationships and power struggles, with the ultimate aim of transcending and challenging these categories. This would disrupt any suggestion of the universality and timelessness of knowledge in that knowledges would always be seen as strategically provisional (Lewis, 1997: 16). These strategies could be viewed in a similar light to Lyotard's 'little narrative' or petit récit, where knowledge is put together locally on a tactical basis with a specific objective in mind by a group of people (Sim, 1998: 8–9).

Perhaps the notion of 'postfeminism' is a useful one, not as popular notions of it as hostile to the feminist project, but as the critical engagement with hegemonic assumptions of second wave feminist epistemologies, informed by understandings of postmodernism, poststructuralism and postcolonialism. Brooks explains it in this way:

> Postfeminism expresses the intersection of feminism with postmodernism, poststructuralism, and post-colonialism, and as such represents a dynamic movement capable of challenging modernist, patriarchal and imperialist frameworks. In the process postfeminism facilitates a broad-based, pluralistic conception of the application of feminism, and addresses the demands of marginalised, diasporic and colonised cultures for a non-hegemonic feminism capable of giving voice to local, indigenous and post-colonial feminisms.
>
> (1997: 4)

This notion of postfeminism could be seen as a fruitful one in the South African context as it could be used to challenge the colonising dominance of Anglo-American second wave feminism, with its implicit ethnocentrism and racism.

Although we must acknowledge that difference has been used to justify inhumane and lethal practices in the apartheid era, I believe contrary to Simone de Beauvoir, who saw it as a contaminated concept which should be abandoned (Braidotti, 1997), that is is possible to 'cleanse' it and that forms of feminist postmodernism can be useful theoretical tools of analysis in the South African context. In examining past social policies, I have suggested why feminist postmodern ideas of 'difference' may have been regarded suspiciously in South Africa, where modernist notions of unity, emancipation and cohesion have been the responses to extreme forms of marginalisation through 'plurality-talk'. As academics and social workers, much work will have to be undertaken to demonstrate the value of feminist postmodern ideas of difference.

Notes

1 I would like to thank the following people who commented on draft versions of this chapter: Brenda Leibowitz, Sharman Wickham, Kathy Collins, Gary Duffield, Anne Knott, Tammy Shefer and Selma Sevenhuijsen.
2 'White', 'coloured', 'Indian' and 'African' are apartheid racial categorisations, but are still utilised as the apartheid legacy has meant that these terms correspond strongly to economic and social status.

Bibliography

Abbot, P. and Wallace, C. (1997) *An Introduction to Sociology: Feminist Perspectives*, 2nd edition, London and New York: Routledge.
Alcoff, L. (1995) 'Cultural feminism versus post-structuralism: the identity crisis in feminist theory', in N. Tuana and R. Tong (eds) *Feminism and Philosophy: Essential Readings in Theory, Reinterpretation and Application*, Boulder, CO: Westview Press.
Alexander, M.J. and Mohanty, C.T. (eds) *Feminist Genealogies, Colonial Legacies, Democratic Futures*, New York and London: Routledge.
Bozalek, V. (1997) 'Gender equality and welfare rights in South Africa: the Lund committee on child and family support', *Women and Human Rights Documentation Centre Community Law Centre*, 1(1): 3–4.
Braidotti, R. (1997) 'Sexual difference theory', in A.M. Jaggar and I.M. Young, *A Companion to Feminist Philosophy*, Oxford: Blackwell.
Brooks, A. (1997) *Postfeminisms: Feminism, Cultural Theory and Cultural Forms*, London: Routledge.
Bundy, C. (1990) 'Land, law and power: forced removals in historical context', in C. Murray and C. O'Regan (eds) *No Place to Rest: Forced Removals and the Law in South Africa*, Cape Town: Oxford University Press.
Burman, E. (1998) 'The child, the woman and the cyborg: (im)possibilities of feminist development psychology', in K. Henwood, C. Griffin and A. Phoenix (eds) *Standpoints and Differences: Essays in the Practice of Feminist Psychology*, London: Sage.
Burman, E., Kottler, A., Levett, A. and Parker, I. (1997) 'Power and discourse: culture and change in South Africa', in A. Levett, A. Kottler, E. Burman and I. Parker (eds) *Culture, Power and Difference: Discourse Analysis in South Africa*, London: Zed Books.
Butler, J. (1990) *Gender Trouble: Feminism and the Subversion of Identity*, London: Routledge.

Davis, D. (1998) 'Let's avoid a new form of intellectual apartheid', *Sunday Times*, 18 October, p. 24.

Department of Social Welfare (1950) *Report of the Department of Social Welfare for the Period 1st October, 1937, to 31st March, 1949, U.G. No. 36-1950*, Pretoria: Government Printer.

Ferguson, K. (1993) *The Man Question: Visions of Subjectivity in Feminist Theory*, Berkeley, CA: University of California Press.

Foucault, M. (1988) 'Politics and reason', in L. Kritzman (ed.) *Michel Foucault: Politics, Philosophy, Culture: Interviews and Other Writings 1977–1984*, trans. A. Sheridan *et al.*, London: Routledge.

Fraser, N. (1989) 'Women, welfare and the politics of need interpretation', in N. Fraser *Unruly Practices: Power, Discourse and Gender in Contemporary Theory*, Cambridge: Polity Press.

Fraser, N. and Nicholson, L. (1990) 'Social criticism without philosophy: an encounter between feminism amd postmodernism', in L. Nicholson (ed.) *Feminism/Postmodernism*, London: Routledge.

Garry, A. and Pearsall, M. (1996) *Women, Knowledge and Reality: Explorations in Feminist Philosophy*, London: Routledge.

Greater Johannesburg Welfare, Social Service and Development Forum (1998) *Submission to the Truth and Reconciliation Commission*, Johannesburg: unpublished.

Haraway, D. (1988) 'Situated knowledges: the science question in feminism and the privilege of partial perspective', *Feminist Studies*, 14(3): 575–99.

Harding, S. (1990) 'Feminism, science and the anti-enlightenment critique', in L. Nicholson (ed.), *Feminism/Postmodernism*, London: Routledge.

Hartsock, N. (1996) 'Postmodernism and political change: issues for feminist theory', in S. Hekman (ed.) *Feminist Interpretations of Michel Foucault*, Pennsylvania: Pennsylvania State University Press.

Harvey, E. (1994) *Social Change and Family Policy in South Africa, 1930 to 1986*, Co-operative Research Programme on Marriage and Family Life, Pretoria: Human Sciences Research Council.

Hekman, S. (ed.) *Feminist Interpretations of Michel Foucault*, Pennsylvania: The Pennsylvania State University Press.

Hirschmann, N.J. and Di Stefano, C. (eds) (1996) *Revisioning the Political: Feminist Reconstructions of Traditional Concepts in Western Political Theory*, Boulder, CO: Westview Press.

Howe, D. (1994) 'Modernity, postmodernity and social work', *British Journal of Social Work* 24(5): 513–32.

Kotze, F. (1996) 'Social welfare policy for a post-apartheid South Africa: a developmental perspective', unpublished PhD dissertation, Cape Town: University of the Western Cape.

Levett, A., Kottler, A., Burman, E. and Parker, I. (eds) (1997) *Culture, Power and Difference: Discourse Analysis in South Africa*, London: Zed Books.

Lewis, D. (1997) 'The challenges of post-colonial theory', unpublished paper delivered at Colloquium in Feminist Theories/Practice, African Gender Institute, University of Cape Town.

Mazibuko, Fikile (1996) 'Social work and sustainable development: the challenges for practice, training and policy in South Africa', paper presented at the Joint World Congress of the International Federation of Social Workers and the International Association of Schools of Social Work, Hong Kong.

Mbeki, T. (1998) *Africa: The Time has Come*, Cape Town: Tafelberg Publishers.

Naidoo, M.T. and Bozalek, V. (1997) 'Maintenance grant parity – women pay the price', *Agenda* 33: 26–32.

Nicholson, L. (ed.) (1990) *Feminism/Postmodernism*, New York and London: Routledge.

O'Brien, M. and Penna, S. (1998) *Theorising Welfare: Enlightenment and Modern Society*, London: Sage.

Parpart, J.L. and Marchand, M.H. (1995) 'Exploding the canon: an introduction/conclusion', in M.H. Marchand and J.L. Parpart (eds) *Feminism/Postmodernism/Development*, London and New York: Routledge.

Parton, N. (1994) 'Problematics of government, (post)modernity and social work', *British Journal of Social Work* 24(1): 9–32.

Ramazanoglu, C. (ed.) (1993) *Up Against Foucault: Explorations of Some Tensions Between Foucault and Feminism*, London and New York: Routledge.

(Republic of South Africa, Department of Social Welfare and Pensions (1966) Circular No. 29 of 166, South African National Council for Child Welfare, Pretoria, Government Printers.)

Republic of South Africa (1996) *The Constitution of the Republic of South Africa Act 108 of 1996*, Wynberg: Constitutional Assembly.

Sim, S. (ed.) (1998) *The Icon Critical Dictionary of Postmodern Thought*, Cambridge: Icon Books.

Smith, C. and White, S. (1997) 'Parton, Howe and postmodernity: a critical comment on mistaken identity', *British Journal of Social Work* 27: 275–95.

Sunde, J. and Bozalek, V. (1995) '(Re)presenting "the family": familist discourses, welfare and the state', *Transformation* 26: 63–77.

Thornham, S. (1998) 'Postmodernism and feminism (or: repairing our own cars)', in S. Sim (ed.) *The Icon Critical Dictionary of Postmodern Thought*, Cambridge: Icon Books.

Wakefield, N. (1990) *Postmodernism: The Twilight of the Real*, London: Pluto Press.

Index